Preparation for the Diplo Royal College Obstetricians Gynaecologists

CW01083781

Janice Rymer MRCOG FRNZCOG
Senior Registrar in Obstetrics and Gynaecology,
Guy's Hospital, London

Gregory Davis MRCOG FRNZCOG
Research Registrar, Department of Obstetrics and Gynaecology,
Guy's Hospital, London

Adam Rodin BSc MRCOG
Senior Registrar in Obstetrics and Gynaecology,
Farnborough Hospital

Michael Chapman MRCOG
Chairman of the Academic Division of Obstetrics and Gynaecology,
United Medical and Dental Schools, University of London

CHURCHILL LIVINGSTONE
EDINBURGH LONDON MELBOURNE AND NEW YORK 1990

CHURCHILL LIVINGSTONE
Medical Division of Longman Group UK Limited

Distributed in the United States of America by Churchill
Livingstone Inc., 650 Avenue of the Americas, New York, N.Y. 10011,
and by associated companies, branches and representatives
throughout the world.

First published 1990
    Reprinted 1993
    Reprinted 1994

ISBN 0-443-04248-9

British Library Cataloguing in Publication Data
A catalogue record for this book is available from the British Library

Library of Congress Cataloging in Publication Data
Preparation and revision for the diploma of the Royal College of
    Obstetricians and Gynaecologists/Janice Rymer . . . [et al.].
        p.   cm.
    Half title: Preparation and revision for the DRCOG.
    ISBN 0-443-04248-9
    1. Gynecology—Examinations, questions, etc.   2. Obstetrics—
—Examinations, questions, etc.   I. Rymer, Janice.   II. Title:
Preparation and revision for the DRCOG.
    [DNLM: 1. Gynecology—examination questions.   2. Obstetrics—
—examination questions.   WP 18 P927]
RG111.P74   1991
618'.076—dc20
DNLM/DLC
for Library of Congress   90-1812
                                                       CIP

The
publisher's
policy is to use
**paper manufactured
from sustainable forests**

Printed in Great Britain by Bookcraft (Bath) Limited

Preface

The Diploma of the Royal College of Obstetricians and Gynaecologists is an examination to establish that a medical practitioner is adequately prepared to undertake Obstetrics and Gynaecology in a general practice setting. This book aims to provide basic knowledge of the syllabus and to assist the candidate to pass the examination. It begins by describing the structure of the examination in detail and devotes a chapter to each section. In these chapters advice on preparation is given and example questions are provided for practice. It is emphasized in the text that the place to learn obstetrics and gynaecology is on the wards, in clinics and in theatre. Discussion with colleagues and background reading is essential in Obstetrics and Gynaecology as there are many areas of controversy.

In covering the syllabus we have aimed for a 'common-sense' approach and have not dealt with minutiae. We have outlined controversial areas and acknowledged that other views exist.

Each chapter commences with a section outlining the 'expectations of the examiners' to provide guidance for the candidate to concentrate on the core of the subject. Our coverage is not definitive and should be augmented with other texts, outlined in 'suggested reading'.

We thank our four contributors for providing their specialist expertise. We are also grateful to Jill Buxton and Roger Jackson from the Royal College of Obstetricians and Gynaecologists who have given us advice about the examination.

Every conception needs a father, and this book has had Dr Joe Rosenthal (General Practitioner) who has painstakingly read and criticized every chapter. He has provided us with excellent consumer critique and we are eternally grateful.

It is our hope that this book will provide the medical practitioner with many of the necessary skills for passing examinations in Obstetrics and Gynaecology, and also a basic knowledge of the subject. We envisage that it will not only appeal to DRCOG candidates, medical students and MRCOG candidates but also have a place in the surgery of the General Practitioner as a ready reference book for common problems.

London 1990   Janice Rymer

Foreword

Increasing recognition of the importance of gynaecology and obstetrics to good general practice necessitated an evolution of the Diploma of the Royal College of Obstetricians & Gynaecologists to fulfil the needs of the enthusiastic GP who wished to declare an especial interest in this aspect of the work. By training in carefully selected appointments and passing a subsequent examination to obtain the diploma, a doctor indicates this to colleagues and patients alike.

Pre-examination courses have been devised. They include a very successful one at Guy's run by the young and enthusiastic team who have subsequently produced this book. Comments from their students have helped shape the text.

It is especially valuable that the lynch-pin of the team is engaged in busy general practice and notable that all the other members are also involved in day to day practice in clinics, labour ward, theatre and wards.

I was, initially, surprised that for postgraduates, instructions concerning examination technique had to be so elementary and so extensive, but I am assured that this is essential if candidates are to do themselves justice. Final medical students, midwives and those sitting other postgraduate examinations will find these sections invaluable especially if they are not used to the United Kingdom system.

The choice of topics reflects the broad range of the syllabus. More to the point, the emphasis given to each relates to its frequency of occurrence and importance in clinical practice rather than as a scoring point in the artificial world of an examination. It is proper that other more complex issues such as assisted conception and control of ovulation are addressed but I was pleased to find the emphasis throughout to be on 'large' rather than 'small' print detail.

Suggestions for further reading are comprehensive but not excessive in numbers. I have enjoyed reading the book and wish the authors well.

E David Morris MD FRCS FRCOG

Contributors

Simon Barton BSc MRCOG
Senior Registrar in Genitourinary Medicine, St. Stephen's and
Westminster Hospitals, London

Michael Chapman MRCOG
Chairman of the Academic Division of Obstetrics and Gynaecology,
United Medical and Dental Schools, University of London

Gregory Davis MRCOG FRNZCOG
Research Registrar, Department of Obstetrics and Gynaecology, Guy's
Hospital, London

Helen Issler MA MRCP
Consultant in Paediatrics, Greenwich District Hospital, London

Ian Page MRCOG
Consultant in Obstetrics and Gynaecology, Royal Army Medical Corps

Adam Rodin BSc MRCOG
Senior Registrar in Obstetrics and Gynaecology, Farnborough Hospital

Jonathan Rosenthal BSc MBBCh DRCOG
General Practitioner

Janice Rymer MRCOG FRNZCOG
Senior Registrar in Obstetrics and Gynaecology, Guy's Hospital, London

Christine Watson MD DRCOG DCH
Senior Clinical Medical Officer in Family Planning and Well Woman
Services, Lewisham and North Southwark Health Authority

Contents

APPENDICES

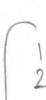

The examination

1. General information

J. Rymer

DIPLOMA OF THE ROYAL COLLEGE OF OBSTETRICIANS AND GYNAECOLOGISTS (DRCOG)

The College awards a diploma to registered medical practitioners who have appropriate postgraduate training and who satisfy the examiners. The diploma is intended to recognize a general practitioner's interest in obstetrics and gynaecology and is not a specialist qualification.

The Royal College of Obstetricians and Gynaecologists produces a booklet entitled *Diploma examination regulations* which can be obtained from the examination secretary. The address is given at the end of this chapter.

ELIGIBILITY

The regulations state that:

1. The candidate must be fully registered as a medical practitioner in the register maintained by the General Medical Council or the Medical Council of Ireland.
2. The candidate must have held a recognized appointment for six consecutive months. (Recognized appointments are limited to the United Kingdom, Republic of Ireland, and HM Forces.)

If you want confirmation of your eligibility, return the form the College send to you in the *Diploma examination regulations* with two certificates confirming your recognized appointment, and your medical registration. The appointment certificate must state that the post is recognized by the College.

Sample certificate

To: Examination Office, RCOG

This is to confirm that Dr. **** has completed to my satisfaction a six

3

month appointment at the above hospital, recognized for the purposes of the Diploma (DRCOG) examination. The post commenced on */*/* and terminated on */*/*.

Signed . . . . FRCOG/MRCOG   Date . . . .

The College can refuse an application and does not have to give the reason for refusal.

If you withdraw your application after the closing date or fail to appear, then you will forfeit the examination fee.

DATES OF THE EXAMINATION

The examinations are held in April/May and October/November. The closing date for applications should be obtained from the college. Late applications are not accepted. The written papers are taken in January and June and can be taken at a centre chosen by the candidate. The locations of the clinicals and vivas are allocated by the College. The entry fee must be sent with the application (in sterling) and the fee is subject to annual review. Details of entry fees are available from the examination secretary.

Recognized appointments for the diploma examination must have been completed by the closing date for the receipt of entries. Evidence of having completed such training must be enclosed with the application.

EXAMINATION FORMAT

The examination is conducted in three parts:

1. *A written paper*. This has two sections: a multiple choice paper lasting 75 minutes and an essay paper lasting 90 minutes, during which two questions are to be answered.
2. *A clinical examination*. You may be presented with an obstetric, gynaecological or family planning patient.
3. *An oral examination (viva)*. This part of the examination may cover any aspects of obstetrics and gynaecology.

You may not attempt the Diploma examination more than five times.

SUBJECT MATTER

The syllabus includes the following topics:

Obstetrics

1. Routine procedures in modern antenatal care
2. Epidemiology of maternal and perinatal morbidity and mortality
3. Complications of early pregnancy
4. Shared care and specialist referral
5. Prepregnancy counselling
6. Prenatal diagnosis
7. Methods of education for pregnancy, childbirth, and the newborn
8. The importance of social and emotional factors in childbearing
9. Antenatal and intrapartum infections
10. The roles of the health care team members
11. The common conditions for which antenatal admission is required
12. The onset of labour
13. Normal labour
14. Pain relief in labour
15. Induction of labour
16. Physiology of uterine activity and oxytocic drugs
17. Fetal heart rate monitoring and acid-base studies
18. Abnormal labour
19. Abnormal presentations
20. Operative deliveries
21. Resuscitation of a shocked patient
22. Breech deliveries
23. Multiple pregnancies
24. Shoulder dystocia
25. The third stage of labour
26. Episiotomies
27. Breast feeding
28. Puerperal infections
29. Puerperal disorders, both physical and psychological
30. Physiology of the normal puerperium
31. Maternal immunization with anti-D
32. Rubella vaccinations
33. Home deliveries
34. Indications for the flying squad.

Neonatal medicine

1. Examination of the newborn
2. Resuscitation of the newborn
3. Common diseases in the newborn infant
4. Normal development of the newborn
5. Congenital abnormalities in the newborn.

Gynaecology

1. Health education and preventive medicine
2. Gynaecological history
3. Gynaecological examination
4. Appropriate gynaecological investigations
5. Congenital abnormalities of the female genital tract
6. Psychosexual problems
7. Infertility
8. Abortions
9. Menstrual disorders
10. Benign lesions of the genital tract
11. Gynaecological malignancies
12. Menopause
13. Urinary tract disorders
14. Vaginal discharge
15. Sexually transmitted diseases
16. Family planning
17. Medical records and clinical audit
18. Communication skills.

The examination time in the DRCOG is equally divided between obstetrics and gynaecology.

RESULTS

Each candidate receives a written result stating whether a pass or fail has been attained. The results are also posted on a board in the College on the day after the final clinical and viva sessions.

Successful candidates are required to pay a registration fee before being granted the Diploma of the Royal College of Obstetricians and Gynaecologists. The amount of the current registration fee is available from the College secretary.

WHEN YOU PASS

Once you have passed, and received your diploma certificate, you are entitled to use the letters DRCOG after your name. The College has a register of diplomates, and you will receive details of College meetings, functions, and events. The College also has limited accommodation which is available to diplomates visiting London. Duplicate certificates cannot be provided in the event of loss or damage.

ADDRESSES

United Kingdom

The Examination Secretary,
The Royal College of Obstetricians and Gynaecologists,
27 Sussex Place,
Regent's Park,
London NW1 4RG
(Telephone London 2625425)

Australia and New Zealand have similar examinations. The regulations can be obtained from the following addresses:

Australia

The Examination Secretary,
The Royal Australian College of Obstetrics and Gynaecologists,
254 Albert Street,
East Melbourne,
Victoria 3002,
Australia

New Zealand

The Examination Secretary,
The Royal New Zealand College of New Zealand Obstetricians and Gynaecologists,
P.O. Box 7148,
Wellington South
New Zealand

2. Preparing for the examination

J. Rymer

The diploma examination is intended for general practitioners who have an interest in obstetrics and gynaecology. It is not a specialist qualification. The examiners will expect a 'common-sense' approach to problems, and management aimed at 'safe' medical practice. To emphasize this we open each chapter in our syllabus section with 'Expectations of the Examiners' to stress what important knowledge is to be acquired. It is very easy to spend time on minutiae when studying for such a broadly based examination as the DRCOG.

The following points are outlined to assist your preparation:

1. The best preparation for the DRCOG is an SHO post on a busy obstetric and gynaecological rotation with teaching from senior staff. Time spent on wards and in clinics is invaluable as the examination is so 'practically' orientated.
2. Ideally, reading should commence before the post starts, and the syllabus in this book provides a good basic knowledge. Thereafter consistent reading around subjects and conditions as they present on the wards will provide the substance of your learning. This is superior to reading a book from cover to cover.
3. It is advisable to plan a reading programme using the College guidelines for the DRCOG syllabus.
4. In all sections of the DRCOG the examiners will ask questions relevant to current practice. They are often particularly interested in current issues that are in the lay as well as the medical press. Therefore it is wise to keep up to date, and this is best achieved by reading the following journals:
   a. British Journal of Obstetrics and Gynaecology
   b. The British Medical Journal
   c. The Lancet
   d. Review articles in the British Journal of Hospital Medicine, Practical Therapeutics, and Hospital Update
   e. Articles in GP orientated journals.
   It is important to form your own opinions about current issues, so that the examiner is assured that you have thought about them.

5. Journal clubs are a painless way of learning, and discussion around the topics is very valuable.
6. Each unit should have organized teaching sessions, and these are very worthwhile, especially if the senior colleagues are present.
7. Writing essays is not a natural ability, no matter how good your knowledge is. It is advisable to practice writing essays, using questions from previous DRCOG examinations and nearer the examination time, restricting oneself to the allocated time. Ideally, a senior colleague should correct these.
8. Revision courses for the DRCOG are good for consolidating knowledge, and for practising skills in vivas and clinical examinations. These are usually advertised at your hospital or in the British Medical Journal. It is important to realize that these courses do not cover the whole syllabus, but are valuable for identifying deficiencies in your knowledge, and allowing controversial areas to be discussed. When you only learn obstetrics and gynaecology in one unit it is easy to miss the fact that certain areas of management are controversial.
9. Senior colleagues have experience and a lot to teach. Listen to them!

3. The written paper

J. Rymer

GENERAL INFORMATION

The written paper consists of a multiple choice question paper lasting 75 minutes, followed by a paper lasting 90 minutes, during which two essay questions are to be answered.

MULTIPLE CHOICE QUESTIONS

The marking system for this examination aims to avoid guessing. A key word, or introductory statement (the stem) is followed by five words or statements (parts) which relate to the stem. The candidate must decide whether each of the five parts is true or false. For each statement correctly answered true or false one mark is given. However, for each statement incorrectly answered, a negative mark is given. If the answer is not known the candidate can mark DK (don't know) on the computer sheet, and no mark is awarded. *This means that if an incorrect guess is made the candidate risks losing a mark, thus negating another answer which he knew was correct.*

The most important advice is to read the stem very carefully. Once you have done this read it again. You are allowed to write on the question booklet so you can mark your answers on it and put a question mark beside those of which you are unsure. You are strongly advised not to guess if you have no idea whether the statements are true or false. It is a mistake to answer every question. 70% would be a clear pass. Therefore if you go through the questions and have answered 90% confidently, it would be best not to answer any more if you are uncertain of the answers, as the negative marking system will work against you.

The first response to a question is more often correct than a later response, so it is unwise to alter the initial answers.

Remember to leave yourself time to complete the answer sheet.

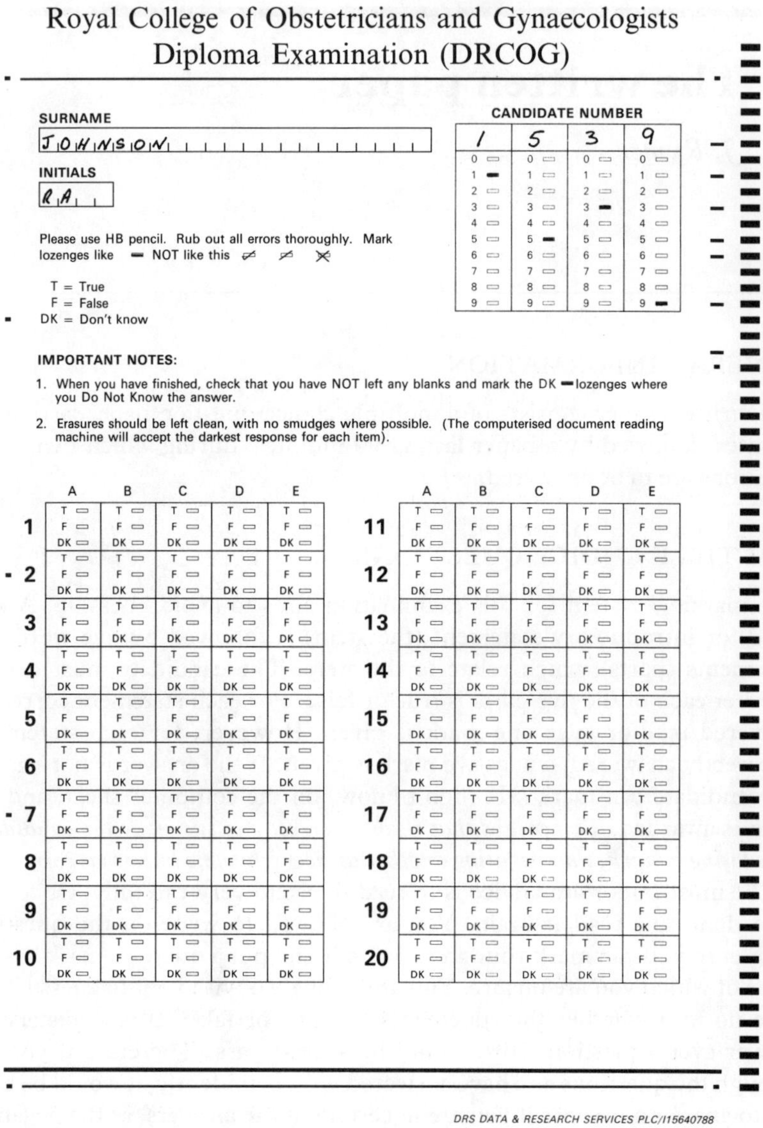

Royal College of Obstetricians and Gynaecologists Diploma Examination (DRCOG)

SURNAME

JOHNSON

INITIALS

R A

Please use HB pencil. Rub out all errors thoroughly. Mark lozenges like ▬ NOT like this ✗ ✗ ✗

T = True
F = False
DK = Don't know

CANDIDATE NUMBER

| 1 | 5 | 3 | 9 |

IMPORTANT NOTES:

1. When you have finished, check that you have NOT left any blanks and mark the DK ▬lozenges where you Do Not Know the answer.

2. Erasures should be left clean, with no smudges where possible. (The computerised document reading machine will accept the darkest response for each item).

Fig. 3.1 An example of a computer answer sheet. It is important to mark T, F or DK for each question.

The following are examples of multiple choice questions:

Obstetrics

1. *In pregnancy*
   A. the plasma volume increases more in singleton than in multiple pregnancies

    B. the blood pressure falls in the second trimester
    C. oxygen consumption rises
    D. the GFR decreases
    E. the fasting blood sugar levels rise.

2. *A raised maternal serum AFP may be associated with*
    A. normal pregnancy
    B. Trisomy 21
    C. threatened abortion
    D. twins
    E. anencephaly.

3. *Rhesus isoimmunization*
    A. does not occur during the first pregnancy
    B. is no longer a problem in England since the introduction of anti-D prophylaxis
    C. may cause fetal ascites in a severely affected case
    D. may lead to Chadwick's sign being detected on ultrasound in early pregnancy
    E. 50 µg of anti-D following a first trimester abortion is sufficient.

4. *The following antenatal complications are more common in multiple than singleton pregnancies:*
    A. premature labour
    B. placenta praevia
    C. congenital abnormalities
    D. polyhydramnios
    E. pre-eclampsia.

5. *Relating to diabetes and pregnancy:*
    A. polyhydramnios complicates 60% of pregnancies in established diabetics
    B. pre-eclampsia is more common in diabetic pregnancies
    C. an IDDM with retinopathy should be advised to avoid pregnancy
    D. the glycosylated haemoglobin level gives an indication of diabetic control over the preceding weeks
    E. congenital abnormality is now the most important contributor to perinatal morbidity and mortality.

6. *A 20-year-old primigravida at 34 weeks presents to the antenatal clinic with a BP of 150/95 mmHg and proteinuria of 4 g/24 hours:*
    A. she should be told to rest in bed at home with the help of a district midwife
    B. a serum urate of 0.45 mmol/l is consistent with severe disease
    C. she may have thrombocytopenia
    D. delivery should always be by LSCS
    E. if she has oedema, the disease will be more severe.

7. *Preterm delivery:*
   A. preterm delivery accounts for 75% of all perinatal deaths
   B. genital infection is not a risk factor
   C. previous preterm labour is not a risk factor
   D. by identifying at risk patients (by risk screening) the incidence of preterm delivery can be reduced
   E. tocolytic drugs delay delivery by a minimum of one week.

8. *The following are associated with a breech presentation:*
   A. placenta praevia
   B. multiple pregnancy
   C. an incidence of 3% at term
   D. Potter's syndrome
   E. Tay–Sach's disease.

9. *Non-stressed antepartum cardiotocography performed at 36 weeks*
   A. can be interpreted using the same criteria as for a pregnancy at 26 weeks
   B. if the rate is 110/minute delivery should be undertaken as soon as possible
   C. deceleration in response to movement is a normal finding
   D. may show uterine activity
   E. if there is reduced variability for 20 minutes the fetus may be sleeping.

10. *The following are appropriate indications for chorionic villus sampling:*
    A. a woman aged 39 with a confirmed 12 weeks' gestation
    B. a woman aged 45 with a confirmed 8 week gestation
    C. a woman who is known to be a translocation carrier
    D. a woman whose son has Niemann–Pick disease
    E. a woman aged 30 whose husband is aged 45.

11. *The following statements relating to vaccination in pregnancy are correct:*
    A. rabies vaccine is safe for use in pregnancy
    B. poliomyelitis vaccination is contraindicated in pregnancy
    C. inadvertent administration of rubella vaccination in pregnancy is an indication for termination
    D. tetanus vaccination carries no risk of intrauterine fetal infection
    E. human varicella zoster immunoglobulin should be given to the term newborn of a mother who has shown evidence of varicella zoster infection in the second trimester.

12. *The following features in a patient's history should alert the obstetrician to the possibility of systemic lupus erythematosus (SLE):*
    A. early onset severe pre-eclampsia
    B. second trimester intrauterine death
    C. early severe intrauterine growth retardation

    D. photosensitive skin rashes

    E. recurrent first trimester abortions.

13. *When a pregnant woman develops hepatitis B*
   A. the course of acute hepatitis B is unaffected by pregnancy
   B. demonstration of hepatitis B e antigen in the mother's serum makes congenital infection unlikely
   C. caesarean delivery is indicated to reduce the risk of viral infection in the newborn
   D. most cases can be managed as outpatients
   E. transmission from mother to baby is commoner amongst Asian than Caucasian patients.

14. *The following statements about oral iron prophylaxis during pregnancy are correct:*
   A. diarrhoea and constipation can occur
   B. if prophylaxis is not given, iron deficiency will develop
   C. non-compliance of the mother occurs in less than 10% of cases
   D. maternal iron prophylaxis is recognized to reduce the incidence of infant iron deficiency anaemia
   E. oral maternal iron prophylaxis is associated with an increase in MCV.

15. *The following statements about severe pre-eclampsia are correct:*
   A. disseminated intravascular coagulation is a recognized underlying cause
   B. epidural anaesthesia is contraindicated if the platelet count is < 100
   C. plasma volume is reduced
   D. diuretics are helpful in management
   E. the serum urate concentration is typically elevated.

16. *A patient at 38 weeks is found on examination, to have a uterine size of 32 weeks. The following ultrasound observations are suggestive of intrauterine growth retardation:*
   A. oligohydramnios
   B. an abdominal circumference on the 50th percentile for 32 weeks
   C. an anterior placenta
   D. a BPD on the 50th percentile for 38 weeks
   E. fetal tachycardia.

17. *Regarding labour:*
   A. induction of labour is not associated with an increased caesarean rate
   B. prolonged labour in a multiparous woman is likely to be due to inefficient uterine action
   C. Kjelland's forceps are associated with an increased incidence of neonatal cerebral irritability

D. the average length of the second stage in a nulliparous patient is 60 minutes
E. the minimum acceptable rate of cervical dilatation in the active phase of labour is 1 cm/hour.

18. *Puerperal psychosis*
    A. occurs in about 1 in 1000 mothers
    B. is characteristically manic in type
    C. usually only results in a two to three weeks' hospital stay
    D. is not recurrent in future pregnancies
    E. is best treated by separation of the mother and the baby because of the risk of infanticide.

19. *Regarding forceps deliveries:*
    A. Wrigley's forceps have a cephalic curve, but no pelvic curve
    B. incorrect application of the forceps can result in cranial nerve palsies
    C. if the station of the head is −1 it is acceptable to use Kjelland's forceps
    D. a pudendal block can be used
    E. the patient does not need to be catheterized.

20. *Postpartum haemorrhage:*
    A. a previous postpartum haemorrhage is a risk factor for a subsequent postpartum haemorrhage
    B. can be prophylactically treated with an intravenous oxytocic with the delivery of the anterior shoulder followed by an intravenous infusion over three hours
    C. is defined as a blood loss of 500 ml within the first 12 hours
    D. can occur with morbid adherence of the placenta
    E. is the main cause of maternal deaths in the latest triennial report.

Statistics

21. *In the Confidential Enquiry into Maternal Deaths (England and Wales) for the period 1982–1984*
    A. hypertensive disease was the commonest cause of direct maternal death
    B. the death rate from ectopic pregnancy had fallen
    C. there was a maternal death rate of 18 per 100 000 total births
    D. about one-third of all maternal deaths were associated with caesarean section
    E. death in association with abortion was included in the true maternal mortality rate.

22. *Concerning the 1982–1984 Maternal Mortality report (above):*
    A. the last report was five years previously

B. anaesthetic causes still claim the most lives
C. direct mortality is lowest in women having their second baby
D. genital sepsis is no longer a major cause of maternal death
E. in deaths due to hypertensive diseases, the cause is usually cerebral haemorrhage, oedema or infarction.

23. *Concerning perinatal mortality in Britain:*
    A. the perinatal mortality rate includes stillbirths and first week neonatal deaths
    B. the three major causes are low birth-weight, malformation and asphyxia
    C. the perinatal death rate decreases with increasing parity
    D. the lowest rate occurs in social class three
    E. if an infant is born before 28 weeks' gestation and shows signs of life, but then dies within the first 24 hours it is not included as a perinatal death.

Neonatal medicine

24. *Babies of diabetic mothers have an increased risk of*
    A. respiratory distress syndrome
    B. intrauterine growth retardation
    C. macrosomia
    D. anaemia
    E. hyperbilirubinaemia.

25. *In herpes neonatorum*
    A. the majority of mothers have a history of herpes genitalis
    B. the herpes simplex virus (HSV) is frequently recovered from the amniotic fluid of infected infants
    C. Type 1 is usually involved
    D. the presence of maternal antibodies is protective
    E. maternal viraemia is characteristically the cause.

26. *The following statements about neonatal resuscitation are correct:*
    A. an apnoeic baby at birth with a heart rate of less than 100 beats/minute should be intubated
    B. in a baby who has been exposed to meconium inhalation it is important to visualize the cords
    C. drying and warming the baby together with simple stimulation normally corrects terminal apnoea
    D. the effects of pethidine given to the mother late in labour may be corrected during resuscitation of the newborn by the administration of naloxone (0.01 mg/kg) via an umbilical vein
    E. a diaphragmatic hernia is a recognized cause of a newborn failing to respond to resuscitation including intermittent positive pressure ventilation.

27. *Congenital cytomegalovirus is:*
    A. present in up to 2% of babies
    B. usual if the mother has a primary infection
    C. rare if the mother is immune prior to pregnancy
    D. usually symptomatic if the virus is recovered from the neonate at birth
    E. characteristically associated with significant neurological impairment following a primary maternal infection.

28. *Recognized complications of preterm birth include*
    A. poor temperature control in the newborn
    B. transient tachypnoea of the newborn
    C. jaundice
    D. meconium aspiration syndrome
    E. apnoeic attacks.

29. *The normal infant delivered at term has:*
    A. a head circumference of 40 cm
    B. an impalpable liver
    C. a plasma glucose above 1.7 mmol/l
    D. brown adipose tissue
    E. no adult haemoglobin.

30. *Regarding fetal circulation:*
    A. the ductus venosus carries blood to the inferior vena cava from the umbilical artery
    B. the ductus arteriosus carries blood from the pulmonary artery to the aorta
    C. the foramen ovale permits blood to pass from the right to the left ventricle
    D. the ductus arteriosus is contractile
    E. the umbilical vein becomes the ligamentum teres of the adult.

Gynaecology

31. *During a normal menstrual cycle*
    A. the proliferative phase of the endometrium follows ovulation
    B. the plasma progesterone concentration rises following ovulation
    C. the average menstrual blood loss is 200 ml
    D. ovulation is dependent upon an intact hypothalamic pituitary portal circulation
    E. the blood loss is normally fluid because of the presence of fibrinolysins.

32. *The climacteric is usually associated with*
    A. a reduction in the level of follicle stimulating hormone
    B. a reduction of circulating oestrogens

    C. an elevated serum 5-hydroxytryptamine level
    D. hyperprolactinaemia
    E. a reduction in the serum cholesterol concentration.

33. *The following statements about colposcopy are correct:*
    A. mild dyskaryosis on a smear should not be referred for colposcopy, but the smear should be repeated indefinitely until a more significant change is detectable
    B. severe dyskaryosis on a smear always indicates CIN III
    C. an 'incomplete' colposcopic assessment can safely be followed by laser ablation providing a biopsy has confirmed CIN
    D. a mosaic pattern suggests intraepithelial dysplasia
    E. prepuberty the transformation zone is more likely to be in the endocervical canal.

34. *The following statements concerning endometrial cancer are correct:*
    A. the risk of developing endometrial cancer is increased in diabetics
    B. postcoital bleeding is the classical symptom
    C. a dilatation and curettage is not required if the colposcopic assessment is normal
    D. the incidence is decreased in nulliparous women
    E. the incidence is increased in women who receive unopposed oestrogen therapy.

35. *Regarding ectopic pregnancies:*
    A. 95% occur in the fallopian tube
    B. PID is the most important aetiological factor
    C. ultrasound should always be performed prior to referral to hospital
    D. bleeding is usually the first symptom
    E. if the pregnancy test is negative the diagnosis is ruled out.

36. *The following investigations should be performed routinely on a woman who presents with symptoms of urinary urgency:*
    A. barium enema
    B. MSU
    C. urodynamics
    D. abdominal X-ray
    E. pelvic examination.

37. *Concerning infertility:*
    A. AIH has been proven to increase the 'take home baby rate' in couples who have unexplained infertility
    B. clomiphene can be given to induce ovulation in anovulatory women
    C. if the postcoital test is normal then a semen sample is not needed
    D. GIFT is used in women who have tubal disease
    E. stress can cause anovulation.

38. *Concerning carcinoma of the cervix:*
    A. the peak age is 50–59 years
    B. it is the commonest malignant tumour of the genital tract
    C. early spread occurs via the venous system
    D. a microinvasive lesion has invaded the stroma to a depth of 3 mm and the lymphatics are involved
    E. it is more common in women who smoke.

39. *Polycystic ovarian syndrome:*
    A. clinical features include hirsutism, anorexia and dysfunctional bleeding
    B. can be treated with clomiphene
    C. LH levels are usually raised
    D. women who have this disorder are at increased risk of endometrial cancer
    E. wedge resection of the ovaries is a common successful form of treatment.

40. *Therapeutic abortion:*
    A. mortality and morbidity increase with increasing gestational age
    B. uterine perforation requires immediate laparotomy
    C. secondary infertility is a recognized late complication of first trimester abortion
    D. the mortality rate of first trimester abortion is less than 1 per 1 000 000
    E. prostaglandins in an asthmatic can cause acute bronchospasm.

41. *Endometriosis*
    A. can be treated with the CO2 laser
    B. can be treated with danazol to create a 'pseudo-pregnancy'
    C. can cause Asherman's syndrome
    D. can cause dyspareunia
    E. if severe can cause infertility.

42. *Hirsutism*
    A. polycystic ovarian syndrome and idiopathic hirsutism account for over 90% of cases
    B. is a side-effect of danazol
    C. is a side-effect of spironolactone
    D. shaving increases hair growth
    E. LH, FSH, and testosterone levels should be measured.

43. *Contraindications to oestrogen replacement therapy for postmenopausal women include*
    A. cervical carcinoma
    B. past history of breast cancer
    C. past history of DVT

    D. diabetes

    E. past history of endometrial cancer.

44. *Infertility:*
    A. the incidence of unexplained infertility in infertile couples is about 10–15%
    B. there is a decline in fecundity with age
    C. if the husband is identified as having 'poor' sperm then investigations in the partner can be abandoned
    D. azoospermia is associated with small testes and a low FSH level
    E. GIFT can be used in women with unexplained infertility.

45. *Genital prolapse*
    A. can be caused by vaginal delivery
    B. vaginal narrowing can occur after colporrhaphy
    C. vaginal hysterectomies have less postoperative morbidity than abdominal hysterectomies if prophylactic antibiotics are used
    D. cannot occur in a nulliparous woman
    E. can become worse after the climacteric.

46. *Hydatidiform mole*
    A. can produce ovarian enlargement and breathlessness
    B. can present with pre-eclampsia before 20 weeks
    C. when complete is totally maternally derived
    D. if partial, has more chance of being followed by choriocarcinoma than a complete mole
    E. can be treated by hysterectomy in the older woman.

47. *The vagina:*
    A. the anterior wall is longer than the posterior wall
    B. the normal epithelium contains mucus secreting glands
    C. is related in its lower third to the bladder base
    D. the pH is acidic during the reproductive phase of life
    E. ovarian function can be assessed by the cytology of vaginal wall smears.

48. *A 25-year-old nulliparous woman is referred from her general practitioner with an abnormal smear:*
    A. a smear should always be repeated before referral
    B. menstruation is the best time to perform colposcopy as the transformation zone is easily seen
    C. ideally ectocervical cells should be seen on the smear
    D. colposcopic assessment may be incomplete
    E. at colposcopy bizarre vessel branching suggests CIN.

49. *Ovarian cancer:*
    A. 30% have metastases beyond the pelvis at the initial diagnosis
    B. can be properly staged using a Pfannenstiel incision

    C. the mortality rate has significantly changed over the past 20 years
    D. laparoscopy is acceptable as a 'second-look' operation
    E. can present with vague symptoms of dyspepsia, tiredness, and abdominal distension.

50. *Dysfunctional uterine bleeding*
    A. is a diagnosis of exclusion
    B. a D and C is therapeutic
    C. the endometrial curettings are abnormal
    D. danazol can be used as treatment
    E. laser ablation of the endometrium is acceptable treatment.

Sexually transmitted diseases

51. *Trichomonas vaginalis*
    A. can be diagnosed by colposcopy
    B. causes clue cells on microscopy
    C. on a wet mount, preparation may reveal motile flagellated protozoa
    D. can be treated with metronidazole
    E. classically produces a thick white discharge.

52. *Regarding AIDS:*
    A. vertical transmission appears to occur in 30–40% of infants delivered to HIV infected women
    B. transmission of HIV to the fetus has been proven to occur in the first trimester
    C. is caused by a retrovirus
    D. nosocomial exposure is an important mode of spread
    E. the diagnosis of HIV in children is difficult due to passive acquisition of maternal HIV antibodies.

53. *Hepatitis B infection in a pregnant woman*
    A. carries a 1.8% chance of mortality
    B. is associated with congenital abnormalities
    C. infection in a pregnant woman carries a 60% increase in preterm delivery
    D. in the third trimester the risk of vertical transmission is 20%
    E. newborns of HBsAg positive mothers should have hepatitis B immunoglobulin at birth.

54. *The lesions of syphilis include*
    A. perivascular inflammation
    B. cranial nerve lesions
    C. aortic aneurysm
    D. vulval ulceration
    E. condylomata acuminata.

Family planning

55. *The combined oral contraceptive pill is protective against*
    A. ovarian cancer
    B. endometrial cancer
    C. cervical cancer
    D. ectopic pregnancy
    E. pelvic inflammatory disease.

56. *Regarding IUCDs:*
    A. menorrhagia is an absolute contraindication
    B. encrustation of a copper device is associated with failure
    C. actinomycoses may be seen with prolonged use of IUCDs
    D. are contraindicated in women who have had a caesarean section
    E. IUCDs inserted within 5 days of unprotected intercourse can act as postcoital contraception

57. *Sterilization:*
    A. the failure rate is 1–5 per 1000 procedures (in females)
    B. vasectomy is safer than female sterilization
    C. in males is deemed successful if two seminal specimens post-operation are 'sperm free'
    D. postoperatively menstrual loss should decrease
    E. the failure rate is increased if performed at the time of abortion.

58. *Regarding the combined oral contraceptive pill:*
    A. it should not be prescribed to women over the age of 37 years
    B. if diarrhoea occurs, the pill may not be absorbed
    C. in higher doses it can be used as the morning after pill
    D. it is associated with an increased incidence of pulmonary embolism
    E. it should not be prescribed in diabetic women.

(answers on pages 32–34)

ESSAY QUESTIONS

There will be two essay questions which are designed not only to assess knowledge but also the ability to communicate in written English and to develop arguments.
An answer consists of 2 components:

1. Knowledge
2. Presentation

They are of equal importance as complete knowledge may be wasted by poor presentation and little knowledge may suffice if well presented.

The following are suggestions for the essay questions:

Dividing the time

Read the instructions at the top of the paper carefully and equally divide the time between the two questions (45 minutes each). For each question allow five minutes for planning and five minutes to summarize. Make sure you have a reliable watch that is synchronized with the clock in the examination room.

Reading the question

Great care is taken in phrasing questions so that ambiguity is avoided. Read the question twice, and ensure that you answer it. Do not pick up on one word in the question and write everything you know on that subject. Answer only what is specifically asked for, e.g. Discuss the management of twins in labour and the puerperium. The examiner does not want to read a detailed account of twins from conception to antenatal care and complications and then just a paragraph on labour. He wants to know about *labour* and *postpartum* management. No credit is given for unrelated facts.

The meaning of various words

A number of common terms used in essay questions have special meanings in this context:

'Describe' means give a full account of, e.g. Describe PID. The examiner would expect a comprehensive account of PID including incidence, pathology, aetiology, symptoms, signs, treatment and prognosis.

'Discuss' means give a selective account of the most important, relevant and controversial aspects of the subject and a comparison of these aspects.

'Diagnosis'. This is not the same as differential diagnosis. If you are asked about the diagnosis of ectopic pregnancy, you should give an account of the steps you would take in order to reach the diagnosis and include the differential diagnosis.

This is best considered under:

1. History
2. Examination
3. Investigations.

'Pathology' includes every investigation that may be undertaken by the pathological department, as well as X-ray pathology, e.g. morbid anatomy, biochemistry, haematology, bacteriology, and radiology.

'Pathogenesis' means the mechanisms of causation, including predisposing factors and pathophysiology.

'Treatment'. This may be subdivided into preventive, curative, and palliative, and may be operative or conservative. Try to answer the questions 'what'? 'why'? 'when'? 'where'? 'how'? Do not forget rehabilitation.

'Complications'. These are usefully subdivided into early, intermediate, and late. They may be considered under various systems of the body.

'Management' means the handling of the patient from the first presentation in casualty or outpatients, to her return to normal health, including rehabilitation and follow-up, i.e. history, examination, investigation, treatment and follow-up.

Planning your answer

Spend a few minutes jotting down your relevant thoughts before starting to write. Then design the structure of your answer. This should consist of:

1. Introduction. The initial paragraph is extremely important. It should introduce the topic and be a preview of your answer. It is useful to begin by defining the terminology and terms of reference for your answer. This eliminates any misinterpretation of the question. In the summary (and introduction) you are conveying to the examiner your general grasp of the topic. Your paragraph should show a greater degree of sophistication than an undergraduate answer. It should not merely consist of a series of definitions derived from the question.
2. Main points to be covered. Divide this section into headings and subheadings.
3. Summary. This must relate to the introductory paragraph.

Set the essay plan out clearly in the answer book and then put a line through it. When the examiner sees a well set out, legible essay plan he will look through it and if most of the points have been covered he will then quickly read the essay, and the mark will probably be favourable. You have placed yourself in a good position because the examiner has immediately seen that you have organized your thoughts.

As you are writing your essay plan it is advisable to refer back to the question to ensure that you are specifically answering the question. The answer must be arranged in a logical and practical order. Mention common things first, as the diploma is concerned with basic knowledge of the subject. If you know rarer things, by all means mention them to demonstrate the extent of your knowledge but do not spend a substantial amount of time on them.

Allow time at the end to read through your answers. Remember that you are under stress and writing quickly, so mistakes may appear. This is particularly the case if a 'no' or 'not' is omitted when trying to make a negative statement.

Layout

The examiner is overworked, bored and tired. He has read many answers to the same question so try and make his task as easy as possible and he will usually look favourably upon what you have written.

1. Write legibly. If your handwriting is bad, practise making it legible. If the examiner cannot read your writing he will not mark the paper. If your writing *is* difficult to read, write on alternate lines.
2. Good grammar and correct spelling are expected.
3. Underline relevant headings and relevant points if it makes the essay easier to read. This will highlight major points so that the examiner can easily see that you have covered them. Numbered headings are often useful.
4. Be brief and to the point.

When you know nothing about the question

You must answer the question. Don't panic. You must still spend the allocated time on this question. Although you may think you know nothing about the subject, remember the following essay structures and you will be able to pass most questions. Some knowledge must be there as you have had six months' postgraduate exposure to obstetrics and gynaecology.

Example 1: Ectopic pregnancy

Incidence
Age
Geographical and racial features
Environmental factors
Predisposing factors
Macroscopical appearance
Microscopical appearance
Natural history of the disease
Spread
Pathological physiology
Management
Prognosis.

Example 2: What are the causes of tubal disease?

Congenital
Acquired
   Physical agents
   Chemical agents
   Inflammation
   Immunological
   Ischaemia

Mechanical
Metabolic
Endocrine
Degenerative
Infiltrative
Neoplastic
Miscellaneous
   Idiopathic
   Iatrogenic
   Psychogenic.

Example 3: Diabetes in pregnancy

Prenatal
First trimester
Second trimester
Third trimester
Labour
Postnatal
Neonatal care
Follow-up
Subsequent pregnancies.

Miscellaneous hints

There are many areas of controversy in obstetrics and gynaecology. If you are aware that there are different schools of thought on a certain subject, acknowledge both, but if appropriate, say what you believe and why. No examiner will fail you for not agreeing with him as long as you can defend your view.

If you know of any new advances in an area then mention them, particularly if you can quote a reference, or have personal experience. The examiner will be delighted to find something new to interest him.

In 'management' questions, think back to what you would have done on the wards or in the clinics. This is what the examiner is after, and don't assume that he knows anything. Everything must be explained in detail. Do not use abbreviations, unless you have them earlier in the text, e.g. cardiotocograph (CTG). After this you can use CTG.

Method of marking

A close marking system is used, and each written question is marked by two examiners. There are five grades of mark:

Grade 5 indicates an excellent postgraduate answer for an entrant to general practice.

Grade 4 indicates a postgraduate pass answer (beyond doubt).
Grade 3 indicates a situation where the examiners disagree as to whether the candidate deserves a pass or fail.
Grade 2 indicates a fail answer (average undergraduate answer).
Grade 1 indicates a fail by any standard.

The examiners are instructed to mark an essay 0 if the answer is totally irrelevant to the question. The chairman of the examination committee will review the answer and report to the examiners.

Examples of essay plans

1. A 53-year-old postmenopausal woman requests HRT. How would you advise her?

Definition of HRT and menopause. Introductory paragraph.
History
   reasons for request
   symptoms
   past history
   family history
   smoking
   medications
   sexual history
Examination
   BP
   breasts
   abdomen
   pelvis
   cervical smear if indicated
Indications
   symptoms
   concern re osteoporosis
Contraindications—history of breast or endometrial cancer
Discuss benefits—relief of symptoms
   adverse effects
      return of menstruation
      tender breasts
Methods of administration
Duration of treatment—controversial
Complications
Summary.

2. An elderly woman presents with urinary incontinence and urgency of micturition. Discuss the possible causes of these complaints and the management of such a patient.

Definition
  urinary incontinence
  urgency of micturition
Introductory paragraph
History of symptoms
  when
  how often
  aggravating factors
  alleviating factors
  associated symptoms
Relevant past history
  previous UTIs
  previous surgery
  past obstetric history
  medical conditions
Social history
Medication—particularly diuretics
Examination
  general state
  abdomen
  pelvic support
  demonstration of incontinence
Investigations
  MSU
  urodynamics
Treatment
  bladder drill
  medication
  physiotherapy
  surgery
Follow-up
Summary.

3. A primigravida, aged 21, has vaginal bleeding in the 32nd week of
   pregnancy. Discuss the management of her case.

Definition
  primigravida
  bleeding
Introductory paragraph
History
  when
  what was she doing at the time
  how much
  associated fluid loss, pain
  fetal movements

Examination
  pulse, blood pressure, general state
  abdomen, fetal heart, fetal lie and presentation
  vaginal—if in hospital do a speculum examination
Treatment—depends on whether continuing or stopped
  Continuing—decision whether to expedite delivery
  Discontinued—observation, maternal and fetal monitoring
Complications
  fetal compromise
  maternal compromise
  rhesus sensitization
  premature labour
  premature delivery of the fetus
Summary.

4. Discuss the management of a primigravida who is found to have a breech
   presentation during the 36th week of her pregnancy.

Introduction re different philosophies on management of breech presentations
Definition—types of breeches
History
  antenatal problems
  past history (especially previous uterine surgery, previous pelvic trauma,
  significant medical problems)
Examination
  height
  general state
  fetal size, position of the legs
  vaginal examination—exclude gross pelvic abnormality
Investigations
  USS
    exclude fetal abnormality
    fetal growth parameters
    liquor volume
  pelvimetry
Management—decide mode of delivery, see weekly
Vaginal delivery
  normal antenatal history
  normal size mother
  average size fetus
  no complications
Abdominal delivery
  footling ± flexed leg breech
  antenatal problems
In labour

 ideally an epidural
 constant fetal monitoring
 obstetrician to deliver
 forceps to the aftercoming head
Summary.

Essay questions for practice

1. Discuss the dangers of obstetric anaesthesia and analgesia.
2. Discuss the value of the postnatal examination.
3. What are the causes of perinatal death? How may the perinatal mortality rate be reduced?
4. A primigravida aged 25 years wishes to have a home delivery. How would you as her general practitioner advise and discuss the relevant issues with her?
5. Discuss the value of blood tests in early pregnancy with particular reference to the immigrant population.
6. Discuss the use of ultrasound in pregnancy.
7. Discuss the differential diagnosis of abdominal pain after the 28th week of pregnancy and before the onset of labour.
8. Discuss the management of jaundice in the newborn.
9. Discuss the management of preterm labour.
10. How may the past obstetric history influence the management of subsequent pregnancy and labour?
11. What is the role of a well woman clinic in general practice?
12. Discuss the management of a girl aged 16 seeking contraceptive advice.
13. Discuss the investigation and management of a patient aged 35 years complaining of irregular vaginal bleeding.
14. Discuss the advantages and risks of intrauterine contraceptive devices.
15. What are the causes of vaginal discharge? Discuss their diagnosis and treatment.
16. Discuss the causes, investigation and treatment of postmenopausal bleeding.
17. At a routine examination of a 30-year-old woman for a cervical smear a pelvic tumour is felt. Discuss the diagnoses and management.
18. Discuss the aetiology and management of dyspareunia.
19. Describe the clinical features and conservative management of endometriosis.
20. Discuss the morbidity associated with contraceptive methods in current use.

Final hints

Read the instructions carefully about where to write your name and candidate number.

 Hand in all your answer papers.

Use commonsense in your answers. The examiners are interested in assuring themselves that you are practical and safe.

ANSWERS TO MULTIPLE CHOICE QUESTIONS

Correct answers

Obstetrics

1. B.C.
2. A.C.D.E.
3. C.E. Rhesus isoimmunization has dramatically decreased in incidence but has by no means disappeared. 'D' is an example of a statement that should not be answered, as most people are not familiar with Chadwick's sign. It is a clinical sign of early pregnancy.
4. A.B.C.D.E. This question emphasizes the fact that nearly all antenatal complications are more common in multiple pregnancies.
5. B.D.E. Polyhydramnios complicates 25% of pregnancies in established diabetics. Diabetic retinopathy, diabetic vascular disease and neuropathy are not adversely affected by pregnancy.
6. B.C.
7. A. There is no evidence that identification of risk factors reduced the incidence of preterm delivery. Tocolysis has not been shown to reduce perinatal morbidity or mortality.
8. A.B.C.D.
9. D.E. At 26 weeks the variability may be reduced. If there are no other adverse features, a fetal heart rate of 110/minute is normal. Decelerations in response to movements are an ominous sign. Fetuses do have sleep cycles of 20 minutes, so a CTG must be continued for longer than 20 minutes to see if it becomes reactive.
10. A.B.C.D.
11. A.D. If vaccination is required in pregnancy, live vaccines should be avoided. Passive immunization is available with anti-rabies human immunoglobulin. The Salk inactivated virus is used for poliomyelitis vaccination in pregnancy.
12. A.B.C.D.E.
13. D.E. Acute maternal infection with hepatitis B virus may result in congenital hepatitis and the risk depends on the trimester in which maternal infection occurs, being highest at term.
14. A.E.
15. B.C.E. Severe pre-eclampsia can result in DIC. As the plasma volume is reduced in these women, diuretics are contraindicated.
16. A.B.
17. C.E. In the active phase of the first stage of labour the cervix dilates at up to 3 cm and 6 cm/hour in primigravidae and multigravidae respectively (the minimum acceptable rate is 1 cm/hour). The average length

of the second stage in primigravidae is 40 minutes, and in multiparae, 20 minutes.

18. A.
19. B.D.
20. A.B.D. A postpartum haemorrhage is defined as a blood loss of ⩾ 500 ml within the first 24 hours after delivery. Hypertensive diseases of pregnancy were the main cause of maternal deaths in the latest triennial report.

Statistics

21. A.B.D.E. For the period 1982–1984, the death rate from ectopic pregnancies has halved, despite an increase in the incidence of ectopic pregnancy. The maternal death rate per 100 000 total births was 8.6.
22. C.D.E. The report on confidential enquiries into maternal deaths in England and Wales is performed every three years.
23. A.B. The perinatal mortality rate is the number of stillbirths and first week deaths occurring from 28 completed weeks of pregnancy to seven days after birth per 1000 total births, but if an infant is born before 28 weeks' gestation and shows signs of life but then dies within seven days, it is to be included as a perinatal death.

Neonatal medicine

24. A.B.C.E. Severe diabetics are at risk of IUGR.
25. A.
26. A.B.D.E.
27. A. CMV is the most common viral infection during pregnancy. By the time an infant is born with the stigmata of congenital CMV infection, damage has occurred in utero and therapy at birth is not effective. There are currently no therapies or immunization practices.
28. A.B.C.E. The passage of meconium is rare in preterm infants, and if it occurs, listeriosis should be thought of.
29. C.D.
30. B.D.E.

Gynaecology

31. B.D.E. The average menstrual blood loss is 30–80 ml.
32. B. FSH and LH levels rise, and oestradiol levels fall.
33. D.E.
34. A.E. Intermenstrual bleeding is the classical symptom of endometrial carcinoma, and postcoital bleeding is suggestive of cervical carcinoma. A postmenopausal woman who has bleeding should be referred for a dilatation and curettage.
35. A.B.

36. B.C.E.
37. B.E.
38. A.E. Cervical cancer is second to ovarian as the commonest malignant tumour of the genital tract. The incidence of cervical cancer has fallen but the peak age is still 50–59 years, and the incidence has doubled in women under 40 years. The lymphatics are not involved in a micro-invasive lesion.
39. B.C.D.
40. A.C.D.E. If uterine perforation occurs during the procedure, a laparoscopy should be performed and the completion of the evacuation performed while another operator is watching through the laparoscope. Laparotomy is carried out if the uterine tear is actively bleeding.
41. A.D.E. Danazol creates a 'pseudo-menopause'.
42. A.B.E. Spironolactone is used in treatment of hirsutism.
43. B.E.
44. A.B.E. It is common in cases of 'infertility' to have 'subfertility' in both partners. Men with azoospermia have small testes and high FSH levels.
45. A.B.C.E.
46. A.B.E. Complete hydatidiform moles are totally paternally derived.
47. D.E.
48. D.E. A smear showing severely dyskaryotic cells demands colposcopic referral and a smear showing malignant cells demands urgent referral.
49. D.E. 75% of women with ovarian carcinoma have stage III or stage IV disease at time of presentation. A vertical incision is essential for correct staging. Laparotomy is usually performed, but laparoscopy is acceptable and this is done at one year postoperatively.
50. A.D.E. A dilatation and curettage is a diagnostic procedure.

Sexually transmitted diseases

51. A.C.D. *Trichomonas* is easily diagnosed by colposcopy and typical Y-shaped vessels are seen. Clue cells are usually associated with *Gardnerella vaginalis*. The classical discharge of *Trichomonas* is usually profuse, offensive, and greenish-yellow.
52. A.B.C.E.
53. A.E. Hepatitis infection in pregnancy is associated with a 20% increase in preterm delivery. In the third trimester the risk of vertical trans-mission is 66% and less than 10% if the virus is acquired earlier.
54. A.B.C.D.

Family planning

55. A.B.D.E.
56. B.C.E. Beware of questions that say 'absolute'.
57. A.B.C.E.
58. B.C.D.

4. The clinical examination

J. Rymer

GENERAL INFORMATION

The College will send you instructions on where your clinical examination is to take place. Allow yourself plenty of time to find the hospital and the ward or clinic where the examinations are being conducted. You should be dressed appropriately. You should take a stethoscope, tape measure, and a pregnancy calculator with you, although they may be provided. When you arrive, introduce yourself to the person who is running the examinations, and they will show you around and go over the time allocation again. If you are unsure of anything, do ask, as they will know all the rules and regulations. Ask the names of your examiners.

Each candidate is given one patient for the clinical examination. The patient may be a gynaecological, a family planning, or an obstetric patient. You are allowed to spend 20 minutes with the patient and during this time you must take a history, examine the patient, test the urine and prepare your presentation. At the end of this time the examiners will enter the room, introduce themselves, and ask you to give a summary of the history, and examination findings. They will then ask you to examine the patient in front of them. Listen carefully to what they ask you to examine as they may be quite specific. They will then take you to another room to ask you more questions about the patient.

The purpose of this part of the examination is to assess your clinical abilities, and to check that you have a good 'bed-side' manner. Always treat the patients as individuals, and be considerate. Never hurt or embarrass the patient, and always be gentle. You want to convey to the examiner that you are a kind, compassionate, and discerning clinician.

In order to prepare for this part of the examination you should take every opportunity to present cases to your registrars or consultants. In a busy clinical job the opportunity arises many times every day.

THE OBSTETRIC CASE

History

The organizer will have told you the patient's name. As soon as you walk in the room, introduce yourself to the patient. It may help to tell her that you are a qualified doctor intending to be a general practitioner and this postgraduate examination is important for your career.

Remember that some patients are excellent historians, and some are not. If there is a language problem, do not panic. The examiners will do no better than you, as they have all been in similar situations. Be a little guarded when patients tell you the results of investigations, or their diagnosis. They may have misunderstood what they have been told.

Ask and record the patient's age, nationality, marital status, and occupation.

A good leading question to take you into the problem is 'How is your pregnancy going?'. The patient should then tell you if there is a problem. It is then important to establish the date of her last menstrual period (LMP). Examiners are obsessed with your accuracy in estimating gestation. Enquire whether her menstrual cycle was regular before conception, or whether she had been on hormonal contraception. Was the gestation confirmed by an early ultrasound scan? Then talk about the specific problem and the relevant facts. Make sure that you enquire specifically about all antenatal admissions, and special investigations. Weight gain should be noted. Enquire whether she has taken any drugs, smoked, or drunk alcohol during the pregnancy. Also ask about any social problems that may have arisen throughout the pregnancy or any problems anticipated after delivery. As this is an examination for general practitioners, examiners will expect a detailed social history, and remember that socioeconomic factors may well have an important influence on pregnancy outcome. Take this opportunity to enquire about the intended mode of infant feeding. She may have a perfectly normal pregnancy.

Details of previous pregnancies in chronological order are essential: how many? Antenatal problems, and length of pregnancies? Labour problems? What type of deliveries? Weight, condition, and sex of babies. Did she breastfeed the babies? Are they still alive and well? Were there any miscarriages, terminations, ectopic or molar pregnancies? Has she changed partners?

Has she ever been in hospital for any other reasons? Has she ever had any gynaecological problems (especially infertility), or surgery of any kind? Enquire about medical or psychiatric illnesses, particularly depression.

Ask her if she knows her rubella status, blood group, and sickle cell status. Is she allergic to any drugs, and did she take any medications before her pregnancy? Is she currently on any medication?

Family history should include any relevant facts concerning the health of parents, siblings, and offspring. Specific enquiry should be made about diabetes, hypertension in pregnancy and any congenital abnormalities.

Social history should include details of marital status, occupations of both partners, and whether they have their own home. Details of how long the patient intends to work for are important, and whether she intends to work after the baby is born.

Smoking, alcohol, and illicit drug ingestion history is important.

General examination

Observe the patient's facies, demeanour, and nutritional state. Ask yourself, 'does the patient look well?'. A pregnant patient should have 'the bloom of pregnancy' due to vasodilation and increased blood volume. Start by looking at the patient's hands. The blood pressure can then be taken, in the semiprone or lateral position. Check the conjunctivae for clinical evidence of anaemia. If the patient is hypertensive remember to examine the optic fundi but do not spend too much time on this aspect. Look for thyroid enlargement, and inspect and palpate the patient's breasts. The heart and lungs should be auscultated. Sacral oedema, and pretibial oedema should be tested for. The legs should be inspected for varicosities, and the reflexes must be tested.

Abdominal examination

As with every medical examination remember: inspection, palpation, percussion and auscultation.

Inspection. Observe any striae gravidarum. Is the swelling symmetrical? Are fetal movements observed? Are there any scars present (particularly look for a laparoscopy scar)?

Palpation. Firstly palpate the height of the fundus and measure the symphysiofundal height with a tape measure. Then feel for the presenting part and determine whether it is engaged or not. (The examiner may ask you to express this in fifths palpable above the brim.) Then feel the rest of the uterus to determine which side the back is on. If you are unable to determine the presentation, don't panic, as in some cases this is very difficult.

Percussion is seldom necessary.

Auscultation. You must listen for the fetal heart in the appropriate place. (You may be asked to demonstrate the fetal heart with the sonicaid.)

Vaginal examination

This is only performed at the examiners' request and is always performed in their presence. (This is very rarely expected in obstetric patients.)

Investigations

There will be facilities available for you to test the urine and this should be performed unless the result is provided for you.

Postnatal cases can be used as obstetric cases.

THE GYNAECOLOGICAL CASE

History

The obstetric patient may be completely normal, however the gynaecological case will usually have a presenting complaint. Therefore you should always begin by asking the patient 'what is the problem that has brought you to see the gynaecologist?'. This will then direct your further history taking. In addition to the history of the presenting illness, the examiners will expect you to have determined:

1. Age of menarche
2. Age of menopause (if relevant)
3. Menstruation: a. regular/irregular b. cycle length, and how many days of bleeding c. how heavy? how painful? d. intermenstrual bleeding?
4. Sexual history: a. any sexual dysfunction? b. contraception c. postcoital bleeding
5. Vaginal discharge or vaginal irritation
6. Urinary habits
7. Bowel habits
8. Past obstetric history
9. Past gynaecological problems
10. General medical and surgical history
11. Current medications
12. Smoking and alcohol history.

Briefly enquire about investigations during her present illness, including ultrasound or X-rays. It is important to ascertain to what extent the symptoms interfere with daily activities.

General examination

Make sure that the patient is comfortable. Take a general look at the patient. Does she look well? Has she a normal body build, and are there any diagnostic facial features? Look at her hands, and then take the blood pressure. Palpate the thyroid gland. A detailed examination of the breasts must be performed, as well as auscultation of the heart and lungs. Remember the patient may be preoperative and it is important that her general physical fitness is assessed.

Abdominal examination

Position the patient carefully so that the head is resting comfortably on a pillow and the abdominal muscles are relaxed.

Make sure the lighting is adequate. The area from the xiphisternum to the symphysis pubis must be exposed, but ensure that the patient is not embarrassed. Follow the same sequence as for obstetric cases:

Inspection. Note the size, shape, symmetry, and movement with respiration. Look for scars, distension, masses, discoloration, rashes, bruising, excoriation, dilated veins, herniae, sinuses or fistulae.

Palpation. Ask the patient if there is any area that hurts. Light palpation should then be carried out looking for tenderness starting away from any painful area. Observe the patient's face. Deep palpation can then be performed looking for deep tenderness and abdominal masses. If you do discover a mass you need to elicit the following features:

1. Position
2. Size
3. Shape
4. Edge
5. Consistency
6. Pulsatile or not?
7. Mobile or fixed?
8. Does it move on respiration?
9. Is it tender?

Don't forget to feel for the liver, spleen, and kidneys, and hernial orifices. Check the lymph nodes.

Percussion. Tympanic or dull?

Auscultation. Normal bowel sounds, or a bruit over a mass.

Vaginal and rectal examinations

These should only be performed at the request of the examiners, and in their presence.

Most organizers will warn you about 5 minutes before the 20 minutes has elapsed. At this stage you should be nearing completion, and you should be organizing your thoughts.

PRESENTATION OF THE CASE TO THE EXAMINERS

The examiners will enter the room, introduce themselves and ask you to present the history and examination findings.

It is important to be brief and to the point. Look the examiners in the eyes and talk with authority. You may refer to your notes, but it is preferable not to read them out.

If the case is an obstetric one your first sentence should involve the following points: name, age, parity, gestation, and the problem (if any). This gives the examiner immediate insight into the case, and if he does daydream while you are presenting he at least has grasped the essential points. An example of an opening sentence is 'Mrs. Smith is a 25-year-old primigravida at 36 weeks' gestation who has been admitted to hospital with the problem of raised blood pressure'. Then go on to present the history of this pregnancy, i.e. LMP, problems in the first, second, and third trimesters, and the current problem. This should be followed by past obstetric and gynaecological histories, other relevant medical and surgical histories, medications, smoking and social history. Then present the findings of your clinical examination. This should include a statement as to whether she looked well or not. Blood pressure and pulse should be stated. Refer to the cardiovascular and respiratory systems, and any other relevant points on general examination. (Listen to the examiners as you may be asked to summarize your general findings, which implies only the positive aspects). When describing the pregnant abdomen present the findings on inspection, palpation, and auscultation. Then summarize by including all the information that you stated in the introductory statement.

If the patient has a gynaecological problem, you should include the following in the introductory statement: name, age, parity, and problem. You should then elaborate on the presenting problem, followed by past gynaecological history, and obstetric history. Other relevant medical and surgical history follows, and medications, smoking history, and social history. The summary statement should be similar to the introductory statement.

After the history has been presented, the examiners will ask you to examine the patient. With an obstetric patient they may say 'examine Mrs. Clark'. In this situation you should start by doing a general examination, and they may interrupt and say, 'just concentrate on the abdomen'. If they say 'show us how you examine Mrs. Clark's abdomen', then only examine her abdomen. You will annoy the examiners if you do not listen to their instructions.

Pelvic examination

You are not expected to examine the vulva or perform a pelvic examination unless the examiners are present. If they ask you to perform a pelvic examination, they may require you to give a running commentary. In this situation you must comment on the negative as well as the positive findings. Respect the patient's modesty at all times.

Depending on the problem you may place the patient in the supine or lateral position. Inspect the vulva first, and then ask the patient to bear down or cough so that you can demonstrate gross prolapse. You will be provided with a variety of specula, and choose the size carefully. When you have inserted the warmed and lubricated speculum comment on the state of the vaginal walls and the cervix, mentioning any abnormalities. A bimanual examination should then follow. Comment on the size, shape, position, and mobility of the uterus, as well as any tenderness. If you feel a mass, confirm whether it is rising into the abdomen or not, and comment on its relation to the uterus and its mobility of fixity. If appropriate, offer to perform a rectal examination. Generally, the examiners will decline.

At the end of the pelvic examination you should thank the patient, and then wash your hands.

The examiners will then usually thank the patient as well, and you will proceed with the examiners to another room where they will question you about the management of the case.

The examiners can ask you about any aspect of the patient, the disease, the management, or the prognosis. They are specifically interested in your assessment of the case and what your management would be. They may not agree with your method of management, but as long as you are logical in your approach and can defend your views, you will pass. You should not argue with the examiners, but don't let the examiners easily dissuade you from your management plan.

Do not be upset if you cannot work out the diagnosis. They are more interested in your approach to a problem rather than actually reaching the right answer. You are expected to manage at a general practitioner's level. Equally, don't be dismayed if the diagnosis seems too easy. Common disorders are used for this examination.

The examiners will tell you when the clinical examination is finished, and you should thank them as you leave the room.

MARKING OF THE CLINICAL EXAMINATION

The examiners do not have access to the marks from your written paper. A close marking system is used as in the written paper.

5. The viva

J. Rymer

GENERAL COMMENTS

It is important to arrive early and to be well presented. Each group of candidates is assembled every 20 minutes and taken into the examination hall. Introduce yourself to the examiners. Sit upright in the chair and keep your hands still. When you are talking to an examiner, look directly at him/her.

The viva is held in the afternoon of the day of your clinical examination. You will be examined by two examiners whom you have not met previously in the clinical examination.

EXAMINATION MATERIALS

On the examination table there may be a small slide projector, instruments, pathological specimens and graphs. All the material should be easily identifiable.

Slides of clinical conditions shown to you on a small screen

These should all be readily recognizable as conditions which you have encountered over the six months of your clinical attachment.

Example: a slide showing procidentia. Once you have identified the condition, the examiners may use this to begin a conversation on uterovaginal prolapse. They may ask about the cause, the symptoms, the management and the prognosis.

Example: face presentation. You may not have seen one in the labour ward but the examiners would expect you to have some understanding of this condition. This conversation could lead on to malpresentations, fetal and pelvic diameters.

Instruments

Do not be frightened by the array of instruments that may be on the examiners desk. You will be familiar with them all and the examiners will expect you to be able to describe the indications for their use, how to use them, and their complications.

Example: Sim's speculum. The examiner may hand you a Sim's speculum and ask you to name the instrument, when you would prefer to use the Sim's rather than the Cuscoe's and then ask you to describe in detail how you use the instrument. In this situation he would expect you to describe how to position the patient, and then give a detailed description of how you insert the speculum, and what you are specifically looking for.

Example: Neville Barnes forceps. The examiner would expect you to have no difficulty in identifying these, and to be able to describe the salient features of the instrument. You may then be asked about the indications, requirements, method of use, and complications.

Cardiotocographs

These may be normal or abnormal. You must know about normal heart rates, assessment of variability, and the various types of decelerations. You may then be asked about your management of the patient.

Partograms

Make sure that you are familiar with the partograms used on your unit as they may be different from the ones the examiner uses. The partogram could easily lead into a discussion on management of primary dystocia, and active management of labour.

Laboratory results

These will be the results of routine investigations. You should be aware of normal values for pregnancy (see Appendix).

Example: hepatitis serology. You may be asked whether the woman is infectious, and if there is any risk to the baby.

Example: FSH level of > 50 Units/litre, LH level > 20 Units/litre. This would indicate that the woman was postmenopausal, and could lead on to the symptoms of the menopause, who should be treated, and what types of HRT you are familiar with.

Pathological specimens

These will generally be gynaecological. If you are shown a 'pot', look at it carefully and describe succinctly what organ or organs it contains, what pathological features it has, and what you think the diagnosis is. Always remember to look at all aspects as the pathology may be on the other side. Use all the clues that you can, e.g. the diagnosis may be written on the pot.

Example: a fallopian tube distended with an ectopic pregnancy. Your response should be something like: 'this is an operative specimen of a fallopian tube. It is distended in the isthmic portion by trophoblastic tissue, and a fetus is present. The diagnosis is an ectopic pregnancy'. The examiner may then ask what symptoms the woman would have had, and how you would make the diagnosis of an ectopic pregnancy.

Contraception items

All these items should be familiar.
Example: a packet of a combined oral contraceptive pill. If you are unfamiliar with the particular packet, state what brand you normally prescribe. You must be able to talk fluently about them, and know their composition.

Miscellaneous objects

The scope is endless.
Examples: cervical spatula, Filshie clip, Hodge pessary, amnihook, scalp clip, pudendal needle.

SUBJECT MATTER OF THE VIVA EXAMINATION

The examiners can ask you anything about obstetrics and gynaecology, and any related subjects. They will not ask trick questions at this level, as they are interested in basic knowledge.

They may ask topical questions. They will never open with a difficult question; their policy is to begin with an easy question and take you further on if you can answer correctly. They may ask difficult questions if you can continue but if you cannot answer these questions it is not usually important as you may have already passed that topic. Never mention topics that you do not know anything about, as the examiners may follow up any new subject matter that you introduce.

When you are asked a question, stop and think before replying.

If you are asked something that you know absolutely nothing about, then say so, and the examiners will move on to another topic. If they begin to talk amongst themselves, listen to what they are saying as they may suddenly involve you.

If you are from overseas and do not have access to a particular facility, tell them if you are not familiar with it and they will be interested to hear how you manage the related problem in your own country.

If you do not understand the question, ask them to repeat it. If you still don't understand the question, ask them politely to rephrase it.

Do not actively waste time. The examiners will be annoyed.

Do not argue with the examiners. Be courteous at all times.

PREPARATION FOR THE VIVA EXAMINATION

Mock vivas are very helpful. Your registrars and consultants should help you with these. The vivas are threatening situations and the more exposure that you have to them, the better. If you do practise with your consultant, you will probably find the college vivas easier, as you will usually not know the examining consultants.

Here are a few things that you should prepare:

1. An obstetric topic. The examiner may say 'what would you like to talk about?'. If you have prepared a topic, this will be straightforward, if not, this may prove difficult. Prepare something simple and non-controversial.
2. A gynaecological topic. As above.
3. A recent obstetric article. The examiner may say 'tell me about a recent article in the literature relating to obstetrics'.
4. A recent gynaecological article.
5. Oral contraceptive pills. You must be able to describe both a combined and a progestogen only pill.
6. The fetal skull. Make sure that you know all the names of the bones and the sutures. Diameters should also be learnt.
7. The bony pelvis. You should be able to name the bones of the pelvis and orientate it correctly. The diameters of the pelvis should be known, and the various different types of pelvis.
8. Management of a postpartum haemorrhage. A very common question, and very important for the general practitioner.
9. Neville–Barnes' forceps. Make sure that you are able to handle them with confidence, and can distinguish them from Wrigley's and Kjelland's forceps.

FINAL HINTS

The examiners want to know what you know, not what you don't know. They want to know that you have a practical knowledge of obstetrics, gynaecology, and family planning, and that you will be safe in the community.

6. Suggested reading

J. Rymer

OBSTETRICS

Beischer N, Mackay E 1986 Obstetrics and the newborn, 2nd edn. Baillière Tindall

Chamberlain G 1981 Perinatal mortality. In Studd J (ed) Progress in obstetrics and gynaecology, vol. 1. Churchill Livingstone, Edinburgh

Chamberlain G 1985 Confidential enquiry into maternal deaths. In Studd J (ed) Progress in obstetrics and gynaecology, vol. 5. Churchill Livingstone, Edinburgh

de Swiet M 1989 Medical disorders in obstetric practice, 2nd edn. Blackwell, Oxford

DHSS (1989) Report on confidential enquiry into maternal deaths in England and Wales 1982–84. HMSO, London

Inch S 1982 Birthrights. Hutchinson, London

Studd J (ed) 1981–90 Progress in obstetrics and gynaecology, vols 1–8. Churchill Livingstone, Edinburgh

Turnbull A, Chamberlain G (eds) 1989 Obstetrics. Churchill Livingstone, Edinburgh

GYNAECOLOGY

Studd J (ed) 1981–90 Progress in obstetrics and gynaecology, vols 1–8. Churchill Livingstone, Edinburgh

Whitehead M 1990 HRT—your questions answered. Churchill Livingstone, Edinburgh

Whitfield C R (ed) 1986 Dewhurst's textbook of obstetrics and gynaecology for postgraduates 4th ed. Blackwell Scientific Publications, Oxford

FAMILY PLANNING

Guillebaud J 1989 Contraception—your questions answered. Churchill Livingstone, Edinburgh

Kleinmann R (ed) 1988 Family planning handbook for doctors, 6th edn. IPPF Medical Publications, London

Loudon N (ed) 1985 Handbook of family planning. Churchill Livingstone, Edinburgh
Handbook of contraceptive practice. DHSS Publications, London

SEXUALLY TRANSMITTED DISEASES

Goldmeir D, Barton S 1987 MCQ's in sexually transmitted diseases. Springer-Verlag, Heidelberg
Holmes K, Mardh P, Sparling P, Weisner P 1984 Sexually transmitted diseases. McGraw-Hill, London
Willcox R, Willcox J 1982 Venereological medicine. Blackwell, Oxford
Youle M, Clarbour J, Wade P, Farthing C 1988 AIDS: Therapeutics in HIV disease. Churchill Livingstone, Edinburgh

PSYCHOSEXUAL MEDICINE

Bancroft J 1989 Human sexuality and its problems, 2nd edn. Churchill Livingstone, Edinburgh
Fairburn G, Dickerson M, Greenwood J 1983 Sexual problems and their management. Churchill Livingstone, Edinburgh

NEONATAL MEDICINE

Gandy G M, Robertson M R C 1987 Lecture notes on neonatology. Blackwell Scientific, Oxford

The syllabus

G. RM

70-220'
Feedback.

FSM, LH.

A. Gynaecology

7. The menstrual cycle

G. Davis

EXPECTATIONS OF THE EXAMINERS

A basic knowledge of the menstrual cycle is essential to the understanding of most gynaecological disorders and hormonal methods of contraception. Examiners will not expect a detailed knowledge of the endocrinology of the menstrual cycle but could ask about the basic principles.

HYPOTHALAMUS–PITUITARY–GONAD (HPG) AXIS

In the fifth month of intrauterine life, primordial follicles in the ovary of the female fetus reach their maximum number (approximately 6–7 million per ovary). From then on, follicles continue to grow and become atretic until the menopause. This process occurs independently of gonadotrophin stimulation and under all physiological circumstances including ovulation, pregnancy and periods of anovulation. As most women ovulate 400–500 times in their life, it is the fate of the vast majority of these follicles to become atretic. Once growth is initiated, follicles progress to the preantral stage of development consisting of an enlarged oocyte surrounded by a membrane, the zona pellucida.

No further development of the follicles occurs until the onset of puberty. At puberty, changes in the sensitivity of the HPG system result in the pulsed secretion of gonadotrophin releasing hormone (GnRH) from the hypothalamus. This in turn causes a similar pulsed release of the gonadotrophins, follicle stimulating hormone (FSH) and luteinizing hormone (LH), from the anterior pituitary. Thereafter, FSH and LH are secreted in pulses every 70–220 minutes depending on the phase of the cycle. This pattern of release is modulated by the steroid feedback on the hypothalamus and pituitary.

Follicular phase

At the beginning of each cycle, FSH stimulates further growth in follicles which have reached a critical stage in their development. In normal cycles, the development of one follicle outstrips the others (dominant follicle). The production of inhibitory factors by the dominant follicle and the falling levels of FSH in the mid-follicular phase lead to atresia in the remaining follicles. As the dominant follicle grows, oestrogen production within the follicle increases dramatically leading to the rising levels of oestradiol seen in the peripheral blood during this phase.

Ovulation

It is these sustained and rising levels of oestradiol in the peripheral circulation which trigger the LH surge from the pituitary which causes ovulation. The mid-cycle surge of LH (and to a lesser extent FSH) stimulates the completion of meiosis in the oocyte and the production of progesterone and prostaglandins in the follicle. The prostaglandins and enzymes activated by the LH/FSH surge free the oocyte from its attachments to the surrounding granulosa cells and cause lysis of the follicular wall to release the oocyte.

Luteal phase

With the release of the ovum, the follicle shrinks and the granulosa cells produce a yellow pigment which gives the corpus luteum its name. The corpus luteum produces all three classes of sex steroids: androgens, oestrogens and progestins, but it is the production of progesterone which distinguishes the luteal from the follicular phase. The massive secretion of progesterone is important in preparing the endometrium for implantation and also suppresses the growth of new follicles past the preantral stage. The lifespan of the corpus luteum is 9–11 days after which it regresses and steroid levels fall unless pregnancy intervenes. Human chorionic gonadotrophin (HCG) from the implanting pregnancy maintains the production of steroids from the corpus luteum until the ninth or tenth week of gestation, by which time placental steroidogenesis is well established.

ENDOMETRIAL CYCLE

Proliferative phase

This corresponds to the follicular phase in the ovary. The most obvious response to oestrogen in the endometrium is cell division (hence the name 'proliferative phase'). Mitosis occurs in both stromal and epithelial cells leading to growth of the glands and thickening of the endometrium from 0.5 mm in the menstrual phase to 3.5–5 mm in height at the end of the proliferative phase.

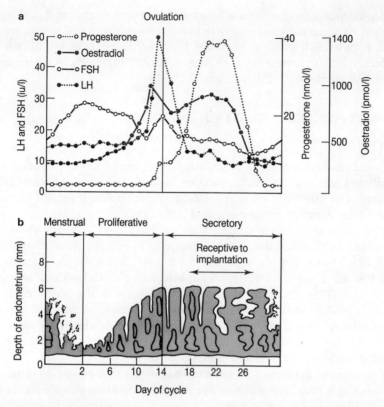

Fig. 7.1 **a**. Hormonal and **b**. endometrial changes during the menstrual cycle.

Secretory phase

The first microscopic sign of a progesterone effect on the endometrium is the appearance in the epithelium lining the glands of vacuoles at the base of cells, displacing the nuclei towards the gland lumen. Mitotic activity ceases but the glands and spiral arterioles continue to grow, becoming progressively more coiled and tortuous. The glandular cells, presumably full of secretory products, bulge into the glands and the glands become dilated with secretory material.

The stroma becomes oedematous in the mid-secretory phase and stromal cells undergo decidualization. They change from being thin fibroblast-like cells to the large polyhedral cells seen in true decidua in pregnancy.

Menstrual phase

Falling levels of oestrogen and progesterone at the end of the secretory phase cause cyclical constriction and dilatation of the spiral arterioles in the endometrium. These spasms are successively more intense and prolonged, leading to generalized vasoconstriction, ischaemia and cell disintegration with release of lysosomal enzymes. Neutrophil leukocytes infiltrate the endometrium and breakdown continues until rising levels of oestrogen in the subsequent menstrual cycle initiate healing.

LOWER GENITAL TRACT CHANGES

Cervix

Cervical changes during the menstrual cycle are of major importance in fertility. Their use to predict ovulation has largely been superseded in the treatment of infertility by more reliable measures but they still form the basis of the symptothermal method of contraception.

The cervical mucus becomes more profuse, fluid and less viscous as oestrogen increases in the follicular phase. Immediately prior to ovulation (2–3 days) when oestrogen peaks, the mucus demonstrates spinnbarkeit which is the capacity to be drawn out into a long thread without losing its continuity. This change is evident as an increase in the pore size of the honeycomb-like appearance of the mucus on scanning electron microscopy and facilitates sperm migration through the cervix. In the luteal phase and under the influence of exogenous progesterone the pore size is decreased and the mucus is less fluid and more viscous.

The changes in cervical mucus can also be observed by drying mucus on a microscopy slide. As ovulation approaches the mucus develops a characteristic 'ferning' pattern in which the dried mucus assumes the appearance of a fern frond. The other observable cervical change is that the os is more open around the time of ovulation which also improves sperm transport.

Vagina

Vaginal secretions are increased in response to oestradiol but the most striking change in the vagina is in the morphology of the vaginal epithelium. Oestradiol stimulates the growth and maturation of superficial cells in the stratified squamous epithelium of the vagina. Therefore, in smears taken from women just prior to ovulation superficial cells are dominant, while more intermediate cells are seen in smears early in the cycle or later in the cycle in the presence of progesterone.

'PHYSIOLOGICAL' TREATMENTS IN GYNAECOLOGY

Infertility

Steroids

Progesterone supplementation to support the luteal phase of the cycle is controversial. It is used on the basis that it helps prepare the endometrium adequately, thereby increasing the chances of successful implantation and reducing subsequent miscarriage.

In women with premature menopause wishing to conceive, sequential oestrogen and then oestrogen and progesterone therapy (mimicking a natural cycle) have been used successfully to prepare the endometrium for the implantation of fertilized donor eggs.

Clomiphene

Clomiphene is thought to have many different actions. As an antioestrogen it binds to oestrogen receptors in the pituitary but does not activate them. This blocks the binding of oestradiol preventing feedback inhibition of FSH secretion. More FSH is therefore secreted by the pituitary producing greater stimulation of the ovarian follicles. A side-effect of this is to increase the incidence of multiple ovulation and subsequently multiple birth.

FSH/LH

An alternative method of inducing ovulation is to bypass the pituitary completely and to give either FSH alone or in combination with LH. Pure FSH is expensive and because the FSH/LH mixture appears to be as effective, the latter (human menopausal gonadotrophins, HMG) is more commonly used.

In this regime, the pituitary may also be bypassed by giving HCG to mimic the LH surge and induce ovulation. LH and HCG are structurally similar but HCG is used as it is cheaper because of the vast quantities excreted by pregnant women.

GnRH

In women who have absent or abnormal hypothalamic GnRH secretion, pulsatile GnRH can be artificially delivered by means of a small, battery-driven pump. This pulsed GnRH allows a normal pituitary–ovarian response and is therefore usually associated with a single dominant follicle and singleton pregnancy.

More recently, synthetic GnRH analogues which have a longer half-life than natural GnRH have been used to abolish a woman's endogenous cycle. These act by initially causing an outpouring of LH and FSH but then down-regulation of the gonadotrophin-secreting cells in the pituitary leads to very low levels of LH and FSH. An artificial cycle is then imposed using LH/FSH and HCG as before. Improved pregnancy rates, particularly in women who have failed to ovulate with other modes of treatment, have been reported using this method. These agents have also been used experimentally in other hormone-dependent conditions such as uterine fibroids, endometriosis, and breast, endometrial and prostatic carcinoma.

Contraception

Hormonal contraception

The two major contraceptive actions of the combined pill are to prevent ovulation and to make the cervical mucus resistant to sperm transport. Ovulation is prevented because the constantly elevated levels of oestrogen and progesterone suppress gonadotrophin secretion, preventing follicle development and the LH surge. The effect on the cervical mucus is a result of progesterone and is the main contraceptive action of the progestin-only pill.

Symptothermal

This method is relatively reliable if practised rigorously and depends principally on the woman detecting ovulation by the increase and change in the cervical mucus.

Irregular bleeding

Anovulatory bleeding

This is a common cause of irregular bleeding particularly at either extreme of a woman's reproductive life. Failure to ovulate leads to prolonged endometrial stimulation and irregular, incomplete shedding. It is treated by replacing the absent cycle regulator, i.e. the corpus luteum, with exogenous progesterone for 7–10 days to achieve endometrial maturation and subsequent shedding after stopping the progesterone.

Prolonged bleeding

Persistent bleeding (not associated with pathology) can be due to a deficiency of progesterone or oestrogen. In the short-term management of this condition, continuous oestrogen, or, more commonly, progesterone will usually stop the bleeding. Following hormone withdrawal, menstruation, often heavy, will ensue. When pathology has been excluded, cyclical therapy for 3–6 months is often necessary to regulate the cycle.

SUMMARY

The menstrual cycle is the product of complex hormonal and target organ interactions. The length of the cycle is regulated by ovarian events, but normal menstruation requires intact functioning of the whole axis: hypothalamus, pituitary, ovary and endometrium. The cyclical production of the steroids from the ovary (follicular/luteal phases) leads to the cyclical changes in the endometrium (proliferative/secretory phases) whose major goal is the preparation of a suitable environment for the implanting embryo.

8. Menstrual disorders

J. Rymer

EXPECTATIONS OF THE EXAMINERS

The candidate will be expected to have a basic knowledge of the physiology of the menstrual cycle. Menstrual disorders are common, and the initial assessment and management of these disorders are within the scope of general practice. However the candidate is also expected to understand what specialist referral will involve and the subsequent management that would occur in hospital.

MENORRHAGIA

Definition

Excessive menstrual bleeding that occurs with regular or irregular cycles.
    Median menstrual blood loss is 30 ml.
    > 80 ml = pathological.

Interesting facts

There has been a tenfold increase in the number of periods that women experience during their reproductive life (reducing family size, early menarche, late menopause).
    If menstrual loss > 60 ml/month, a negative iron balance will develop on a normal Western diet.

Pathophysiology

Menstrual bleeding can be ovulatory or anovulatory. In general, regular, painful periods are associated with ovulation, and irregular, painless periods with anovulation. The latter is more common in the extremes of menstrual life. There is now evidence that in women with proven menorrhagia, there are elevated levels of prostaglandins in the endometrium, and these women have an altered responsiveness to the vasodilator PGE2. Progesterone inhibits prostaglandin production and oestradiol increases prostaglandin production. Ovulatory bleeding is associated with normal levels of hormones, so it is thought that altered prostaglandin synthesis is responsible for the increased menstrual loss, and in particular the ratio of PGE2 and prostacyclin to PGF2α, the former causing vasodilatation and inhibition of platelet aggregation and the latter promoting vasoconstriction and platelet aggregation.

In anovulatory cycles, oestrogen and progesterone levels are abnormal, causing irregular shedding of the endometrium.

Aetiology

1. Physiological, i.e. normal loss but interpreted as excessive. This commonly occurs in women who stop the oral contraceptive pill. Having been used to painless, light periods while taking the pill, they then revert to normal periods which are more painful, and heavier.
2. Dysfunctional uterine bleeding (hormonal). This is a diagnosis which is made after pelvic pathology has been excluded.
3. Congenital, e.g. increased endometrial surface area of which an example is a bicornuate uterus.
4. Traumatic, e.g. IUCD
5. Infective, e.g. chronic pelvic inflammatory disease
6. Neoplastic, e.g. fibroids
7. Metabolic, e.g. thyroid dysfunction
8. Psychological factors
9. Endometriosis
10. Blood dyscrasias
11. Iatrogenic, e.g. drug ingestion as seen in women on long-term anti-coagulation.

'Physiological' and 'dysfunctional uterine bleeding' account for 50% of all cases of menorrhagia.

Assessment

History is notoriously inaccurate but it is essential to distinguish menstrual bleeding from non-menstrual bleeding. The number of pads/tampons used does not equal amount lost, and history of flooding or clots is unreliable. Objective measurement is impractical. Therefore, the diagnosis is based on the patient's own assessment of her menstrual loss.

Examination should include measurement of weight, a search for signs of endocrine disturbance, and a pelvic examination, including a cervical smear if indicated.

Investigations

1. Full blood count: if the menorrhagia is significant then anaemia will be present.

2. Thyroid function tests.
3. Further tests are determined by history and examination, e.g. clotting disorders—clotting profiles, pelvic infection—endocervical swabs.
4. Endometrial biopsy. This should be performed if the menorrhagia is a recent phenomena, if the woman is over 35 years of age, or if there is any intermenstrual bleeding. There are various techniques available. The most common is a dilatation and curettage which is usually performed as an inpatient procedure under general anaesthetic, although a paracervical block can be used. This procedure is diagnostic, not therapeutic although some women experience a few months of lighter periods after a formal dilatation and curettage. A Vabra curettage can be performed in the outpatient's department using a small metal cannula attached to suction. Smaller plastic devices are being introduced with good results, e.g. Gynocheck.

Treatment

Any pathology that is found should be appropriately treated. One is then left with the treatment of dysfunctional uterine bleeding.

Anovulatory

In adolescents, the oral contraceptive pill can be prescribed, making the periods lighter, regular, and less painful. Cyclical progestogens, (e.g. medroxyprogesterone acetate 10 mg daily for 10 days) can be used to induce regular withdrawal bleeds. Likewise, in perimenopausal women, once the endometrium has been sampled, cyclical progestogens can also be used to induce regular withdrawal bleeding. If no withdrawal bleeding occurs, then there has been no oestrogenic stimulation of the endometrium which indicates failed ovarian function, and the 'menopause' has occurred. If the woman is experiencing climacteric symptoms with menorrhagia then it is acceptable to put her on hormone replacement therapy, remembering that she needs progestogens for at least 12 days of each calendar month.

Acute arrest for heavy bleeding. Start with a high dose of medroxy-progesterone acetate or norethisterone and decrease, e.g. norethisterone 30 mg b.d. for 3 days, 20 mg b.d. for 3 days, 10 mg b.d. for 3 days, 5 mg b.d. for 10 days. This will be followed by a withdrawal bleed.

Ovulatory

1. Nonsteroidal anti-inflammatory drugs: These inhibit biosynthesis of the prostaglandins, and reduce menstrual flow in up to 80% of women *if* blood loss is greater than 80 ml. The advantage of this treatment is that pills are only taken for a few days of each cycle, i.e. during menstruation.

2. Oral contraceptive pill: The absolute contraindications must be ruled out, and the relative contraindications considered. Ovulation is suppressed, and the oestrogen levels remain constant. This inhibits endometrial growth producing a reduced menstrual loss.
3. Danazol: The mechanism is uncertain but it induces atrophy of the endometrium as a result of low levels of circulating sex steroids. Normal dose is 200 mg daily. Disadvantages are that it requires daily dosage and has side-effects, e.g. weight gain, virilizing effects.
4. Antifibrinolytic drugs: These probably act by reducing enhanced fibrinolytic activity found in the uterus in women with excessive menstrual blood loss. Side-effects are common, e.g. nausea and dizziness.
5. Hysterectomy: This is the definitive treatment but involves the risks associated with major pelvic surgery, e.g. pelvic thrombosis. Controlled trials have shown that postoperative psychological morbidity is similar to that seen preoperatively.
6. Endometrial ablation: This method is currently being studied. The endometrium is visualized hysteroscopically and destroyed with the laser or resectoscope.

SUMMARY

Menorrhagia is a common symptom which is difficult to assess objectively. As a generalization, heavy irregular bleeding is anovulatory and occurs in the extremes of reproductive life, and heavy regular bleeding is usually ovulatory. In dysfunctional uterine bleeding, hysterectomy should only be considered after failure of conservative medical treatment.

DYSMENORRHOEA

PRIMARY

Definition

Painful periods for which no organic or psychological cause can be found.

Pathophysiology

There is an abnormally high production of endometrial prostaglandins which cause excessive uterine contractions. Generally associated with ovulatory cycles.

Assessment

History is important, as pain occurs with onset of menstruation and then declines. Examination must exclude obvious pathology.

Investigation

If diagnosis is made on history then no further investigation is needed. If treatment fails to improve symptoms then a laparoscopy is needed to exclude pathology.

Treatment

1. Nonsteroidal anti-inflammatory agents are prostaglandin synthetase inhibitors and will decrease pain and reduce menstrual loss.
2. Oral contraceptive pill will inhibit ovulation. Primary dysmenorrhoea is usually associated with ovulation, thus the pill will relieve primary dysmenorrhoea.

SECONDARY

Definition

Painful periods where an organic or psychosexual cause can be found.

Aetiology

1. Pelvic inflammatory disease
2. Endometriosis
3. Ovarian tumour
4. Previous pelvic or abdominal surgery
5. Misplaced IUCD
6. Past history of sexual abuse
7. Other psychological problems.

Assessment

History is important and may take time if psychosexual problems are present. Pelvic examination must be performed, and swabs taken if indicated. Restricted mobility or fixed retroversion of the uterus suggests the presence of adhesions secondary to endometriosis, pelvic inflammatory disease or previous surgery.

Investigations

These will be guided by history, but laparoscopy is indicated in most cases.

Treatment

This depends on the cause. Often reassurance that the pelvis is normal is treatment in itself.

AMENORRHOEA

PRIMARY

Definition

No menstruation by 14 years with growth failure or absence of secondary sexual characteristics, i.e. breast development and pubic hair growth. No menstruation by 16 years when growth and sexual development are normal.

SECONDARY

Definition

Absence of menses for six months (or six cycles) in a previously menstruating woman.

Aetiology

The causes can be divided into compartments:

1. Target organ and outflow tract dysfunction
2. Gonadal failure
3. Pituitary dysfunction
4. Hypothalamic dysfunction
5. Thyroid or adrenal dysfunction.

Assessment

The history should involve specific questioning of galactorrhoea, weight change, hirsutism, life crisis, possibility of pregnancy, recent gynaecological surgery, and cyclical pain.

Investigations

1. Serum prolactin level (× 2)
2. Thyroid function tests if indicated
3. FSH/LH levels
4. Karyotype if phenotype abnormal
5. Ultrasound scan of pelvis.

Treatment

See Figure 8.1. If prolactin level high then refer to specialist centre for CT scan of pituitary fossa and bromocriptine if a microadenoma is present.

Thyroid disease should be treated appropriately.

If both thyroid and prolactin levels are normal, then specialist referral

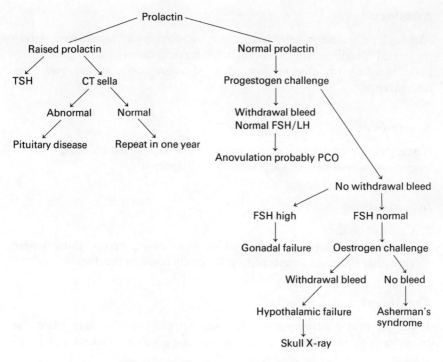

Fig. 8.1   Amenorrhoea—management plan.

would be appropriate at this stage. Management will involve a progestogen challenge test, e.g. 5 mg medroxyprogesterone acetate b.d. for five days. If this is followed by a withdrawal bleed, then anovulation is the diagnosis, most likely secondary to polycystic ovarian disease. In the absence of a withdrawal bleed, a raised FSH level indicates gonadal failure (i.e. menopause). If FSH is normal then an oestrogen challenge test is performed, e.g. 2.5 mg conjugated oestrogens daily for 21 days, with the above medroxyprogesterone acetate regimen for the last five days. If there is no withdrawal bleed, then there is an outflow tract disorder, i.e. Asherman's Syndrome, or cervical stenosis (assuming that the rest of the genital tract has been adequately examined and found to be normal). If there is a withdrawal bleed, then the problem is hypothalamic, but a skull X-ray is performed to check the pituitary fossa.

INTERMENSTRUAL BLEEDING

Definition

Vaginal bleeding occurring in between menstruation.

Aetiology

Although classically associated with endometrial carcinoma, intermenstrual bleeding may also occur with cervical carcinoma. Regular midcycle bleeding or spotting can occur spontaneously on the oral contraceptive pill.

Assessment

History is important, as a recent onset of intermenstrual bleeding is more suspicious of endometrial carcinoma (see Chapter 10).

Investigations

1. Cervical smear.
2. Endometrial biopsy is indicated in most cases, except those where adjusting the oral contraceptive pill rapidly corrects the disturbance.

Treatment

If on the oral contraceptive pill, take two pills on the days when the breakthrough bleeding is occurring, or change to a different pill preparation.

POSTCOITAL BLEEDING

This is the classical symptom of cervical carcinoma.

9. Endometriosis, dyspareunia and pelvic pain

G. Davis

ENDOMETRIOSIS

Expectations of the examiners

Because endometriosis is a common condition which causes pain and infertility, the examiners will expect the candidate to have a sound knowledge of its presentation and methods of treatment.

Definition

The presence of functioning endometrial tissue outside the uterine cavity. Histopathological examination must confirm the presence of glands and stroma.

Interesting facts

The reported incidence of endometriosis varies widely but is probably about 10% of menstruating white women and 30% of women presenting with infertility. It may be asymptomatic and an incidental finding at abdominal surgery for other reasons, or it may cause severe, chronic pelvic pain. The severity of the pain may often be disproportionate to the extent of the disease.

Endometriosis may be present outside the uterus or within the myometrium (adenomyosis) but not usually both. This suggests that the two have different underlying causes. Adenomyosis is a histological diagnosis made after hysterectomy, usually for menorrhagia, and will not be discussed further. Conventionally, endometriosis has been described as presenting in infertile white women aged between 30 and 45 years of higher socioeconomic status. As the use of laparoscopy has become more widespread, this description has become less accurate. Users of the combined oral contraceptive pill have a lower incidence of endometriosis.

Pathophysiology

Aetiology

Classically there are three theories concerning the pathogenesis of endometriosis:

1. *Retrograde menstruation.* Viable fragments of endometrium are known to reach the pelvic cavity during menstruation. In susceptible individuals these may implant leading to intrapelvic distribution of endometrial deposits. This theory does not explain the development of endometriosis at distant sites.
2. *Lymphatic or vascular spread.* Small, viable endometrial 'emboli' can be recovered from the lungs and provide an adequate explanation for the presence of endometriosis at peripheral sites.
3. *Metaplasia of coelomic epithelium.* It is proposed that the repeated inflammatory insult of menstrual fluid may lead to a redifferentiation of the primitive coelomic epithelium which comprises the visceral peritoneum.

No single theory adequately explains the distribution of endometriosis and it is likely to be a combination of the above factors. It is not known what determines a woman's susceptibility to developing endometriosis but it is probably a result of immunological and physical components. In addition, direct 'inoculation' may occur during surgery leading to the development of endometriosis in hysterotomy, hysterectomy and caesarean section scars.

Site

Endometriosis commonly occurs in the dependent part of the pelvis: ovaries, uterosacral ligaments, pouch of Douglas. It is less commonly seen on other peritoneal surfaces of the abdominal cavity, in the umbilicus or scars from abdominal surgery, and in the bowel and bladder. It has also been described in distant sites, e.g. lung, thigh, vulva.

Pathology

Commonly endometriotic deposits consist of multiple small (< 1 cm), raised blue-black nodules which appear as if ink has been injected under the peritoneum. In more severe disease the nodules may be larger with variable amounts of surrounding fibrosis. If the ovary becomes involved then an endometrioma (or chocolate cyst) may form. In chronic endometriosis there is extensive pelvic damage due to fibrosis and adhesion formation.

Microscopically, glands and stroma are present together with a variable amount of bleeding and fibrosis. These deposits may be out of phase with the woman's menstrual cycle but decidualize during pregnancy like normal endometrium.

Assessment

Women may present with symptoms due to the local effects of endometriosis or through the complications that have occurred as a result of the disease. Forty per cent of women with endometriosis present with the combination of dysmenorrhea, dyspareunia and infertility.

History

Pain. Classically, endometriosis is associated with secondary dysmenorrhea. The pelvic pain is directly related to the onset and duration of the menses and is usually progressive unless treated.

Dyspareunia. Intercourse may be painful on deep penetration throughout the menstrual cycle. (See section on dyspareunia.)

Complications.

Infertility. Endometriosis may cause infertility in the absence of other symptoms. Minimal disease is associated with infertility but does not 'cause' the infertility itself as pregnancy rates are the same with and without treatment. More severe disease associated with adhesion formation and pelvic distortion prevents successful fertilization and implantation.

Lower genital tract. Uncommonly deposits in the vagina or vulva may give rise to bleeding or dyspareunia.

Bowel. Endometriosis involving the bowel may cause cyclical rectal bleeding, stricture or rarely obstruction.

Bladder. The bladder is rarely affected but cyclical haematuria may occur if it is involved.

Abdominal wall. Deposits in the umbilicus or abdominal wounds cause cyclical swelling and pain at the affected site.

Examination

Abdominal examination may reveal the presence of a mass (endometrioma) but more commonly there is tenderness in the lower abdomen. Abdominal wall deposits are usually tender and the diagnosis is made on the history and histology after excision. Pelvic examination may reveal nodules in the vagina which can bleed. On bimanual examination the uterus may be tender and fixed in retroversion by adhesions, and nodules on the uterosacral ligaments may be palpable.

Investigations

The diagnosis is usually confirmed by laparoscopy. Involvement of other systems is investigated in the appropriate manner, e.g. cystoscopy and biopsy if bladder involvement is suspected. The extent of the disease is usually classified as mild (minimal), moderate or severe. The American

Fertility Society has produced a scoring system to assess the severity based on the size and extent of the lesions and the amount of adhesion formation.

Treatment

Minimal disease should only be treated if pain is a problem. The treatment of asymptomatic women with infertility is controversial as treatment does not improve their chances of future pregnancy. Symptomatic or severe disease can be treated medically or surgically.

Medical

Medical treatment is based on the prolonged inhibition of ovulation and was introduced because of the improvement in endometriosis that supposedly occurs during pregnancy. It is suppressive rather than curative.

Danazol 200–800 mg/day for 6–9 months. The actions of danazol are complex and it primarily prevents the mid-cycle surge of gonadotrophins. It is an androgen derivative and produces a high androgen, low oestrogen environment which does not support the growth of endometriosis. Side effects occur in 80% of women and are a result of 1. low oestrogen: decreased breast size, hot flushes, vaginitis; or 2. high androgen: acne, oily skin, weight gain, hirsutism. Only 10% of women find the side-effects sufficiently troublesome to stop the drug but it should be stopped immediately if there is any deepening of the voice as this is irreversible.

Combined oral contraceptive. This is given continuously for 6–9 months. Weight gain is a more prominent side-effect than when the pill is given cyclically, but otherwise the side-effects are similar.

Medroxyprogesterone acetate. 30 mg/day is as effective as danazol, is cheaper and has fewer side-effects. Breakthrough bleeding is a common problem which is treated with a 7-day course of oestrogen (ethinyl oestradiol 10 µg/day).

LHRH agonist. Long-acting agonist delivered intranasally or subcutaneously is as effective as danazol or medroxyprogesterone acetate in suppressing the disease. Because of cost it should only be used as a third choice. LHRH agonists lead to very low levels of oestrogen and the long-term effects on bone are uncertain.

Surgical

This is the only means of removing the disease.

Laparoscopic. Small lesions can be destroyed and fine adhesions divided by laser and/or mechanical means.

Laparotomy. Definitive surgery is required for the treatment of severe disease. The object of surgery is to restore normal anatomy and to remove as much endometriosis as possible. The only cure is the resection of all deposits and hysterectomy and bilateral salpingo-oophorectomy. Many surgeons use medical treatment prior to surgery to improve the resectability of the lesions. Hormone replacement therapy can be used postoperatively with a minimal risk of growth in residual endometriosis.

Follow-up

Medical therapy

This is usually effective in treating pain, particularly with minimal disease, but 40% of women will get a recurrence of symptoms at some time after treatment stops. Pregnancy rates of 50–75% are reported in both the groups treated and those untreated.

Surgery

The recurrence rate after adequate surgery is less than 20%. Postoperative fertility is related to the severity of the disease with 60% conceiving after surgery for moderate disease compared to 35% for severe disease. Fertility is greatest in the first year after surgery and conception is unlikely after two years. After this time, assisted conception techniques should be considered.

DYSPAREUNIA

Expectations of the examiners

This is a common symptom which is usually managed by general practitioners without referral to a gynaecologist. The candidate must have an understanding of the physical causes, their diagnosis and the management of this condition.

Definition

Painful or difficult intercourse. It may be divided into: 1. superficial: pain at the onset of penetration; or 2. deep: pain during or after penetration has occurred.

Interesting facts

Dyspareunia is a common symptom but many women are reluctant to talk about it. Often it must be elicited and there may be a combination of physical and psychological factors causing the pain. Pain due to a physical problem often leads to fear of intercourse which exacerbates the symptoms and this cycle may continue after the physical problem is cured. Both the physical and psychological aspects should be addressed if the symptom is to resolve.

Table 9.1   Causes of superficial dyspareunia.

Vulva	Vulvitis
	Atrophic
	Infective (candida, herpes)
	Bartholinitis
	Dystrophy
	Neoplasm
Vagina	Vaginismus
	Vaginitis
	Atrophic
	Infective
	Anatomical
	Vaginal atresia
	Imperforate hymen
	Contracture
	Atrophy
	Postsurgery
	Postradiotherapy
Urethra	Urethritis
	Urethral caruncle
	Urethral diverticulum

Pathophysiology

Superficial dyspareunia may be caused by any of the conditions listed in Table 9.1.

Any pelvic pathology may cause deep dyspareunia but the common causes are:

1. PID
2. Endometriosis
3. Ectopic pregnancy
4. Chronic pelvic pain syndrome (see below)
5. Ovarian neoplasm, e.g. bleed into cyst.

Uterine prolapse and retroversion are commonly listed as causes but are unlikely to result in significant dyspareunia except where the uterus is affected by other pathology, e.g. endometriosis.

Assessment

History

The onset and relationship of the pain to the woman's life events and menstrual cycle are important. The menstrual, contraceptive and obstetric history should be obtained in detail and a full sexual history taken. It is important to assess the woman's attitude to sex and the family history of attitudes to pain and sex. Acute dyspareunia suggests an organic cause, while chronic superficial dyspareunia is more suggestive of psychosexual dysfunction.

Examination

A very careful pelvic examination should be performed to exclude physical causes. The woman's attitude to the examination may reflect her underlying attitude to her sexuality (or a physical problem).

Investigations

Vaginal and endocervical swabs should be taken if indicated. Deep dyspareunia usually requires laparoscopy to make a diagnosis if a cause is not apparent on examination.

Treatment

Superficial

If the cause is organic, this is usually apparent on examination and should be appropriately treated. Vaginismus ± other psychosexual dysfunction is usually treated with vaginal dilators combined with psychosexual counselling. This should be undertaken by a person with experience in this field.

Deep dyspareunia

Any organic cause should be treated appropriately. Unexplained or untreatable disease (e.g. due to previous surgery) may be improved by limiting penetration through the couple using alternative positions during intercourse.

Follow-up

The treatment of physical disease causing superficial dyspareunia is usually successful provided that the woman has a supportive sexual partner. The outcome of psychosexual treatment is variable but pure vaginismus can be effectively cured. The results of treatment of deep dyspareunia depend on the underlying cause. If no cause is found then it may become a chronic problem.

PELVIC PAIN

Expectations of the examiners

Pelvic pain is a common gynaecological problem and the candidate must understand how to approach the problem, exclude organic disease and deal effectively with the psychological aspects of this symptom.

Definition

Pain is localized to the pelvis but it may include lower abdominal and lower back pain.

Interesting facts

Twenty-five per cent of women referred to gynaecology outpatients complain of pelvic pain. The non-gynaecological causes include bowel (e.g. appendicitis, diverticulitis) or urinary tract disease (e.g. UTI, ureteric calculus) and rarely spinal disease. In 30% of patients with pelvic pain no cause can be found at laparoscopy and these patients are characterized as having chronic pelvic pain (syndrome). Malignant gynaecological tumours may present with lower abdominal or pelvic discomfort. Significant pain is usually a late feature of advanced gynaecological malignancy.

Pathophysiology

All nerves from the pelvic organs ascend to the T10-L1 spinal segments but the pain is poorly localized and may be referred to the appropriate dermatome. The cause of the pain is unclear—acute distension of the fallopian tubes or ovaries causes pain (e.g. ectopic pregnancy) but chronic slow swelling may be asymptomatic (e.g. dermoid cyst). Venous congestion of the pelvis causing pain is a controversial issue and unresolved at present. Venous congestion is often striking in acute pelvic inflammatory disease although whether this is the source of the pain is unknown. Dysmenorrhea is caused by prostaglandin-induced myometrial contractions and anything that stimulates uterine contractions will cause pain (e.g. labour, incomplete abortion).

Assessment

History

A full history is fundamental in dealing with pelvic pain adequately and the pain should be defined as accurately as possible:

1. Site and radiation of pain
2. Character of pain (sharp, dull)
3. Duration and nature of onset
4. Periodicity of pain (constant, intermittent)
5. Severity of pain (e.g. effect on sleep, work, leisure)

6. Relationship to menstruation, food, movement, coitus, defaecation, micturition, posture
7. Any alleviating factors and effect of analgesics.

A full sexual history and a detailed social history focusing on stressful life events and current circumstances must be taken. While taking the history, an assessment of the woman's psychological status including mood and level of anxiety should be made.

Examination

A careful general and abdominal examination must be performed. If the pain is well localized, an organic cause is more likely. Similarly, abdominal guarding and rebound are unlikely to be elicited without underlying pathology. Gynaecological pain is usually most severe suprapubically. After speculum examination has been performed to exclude abnormality, a bimanual examination should be undertaken.

Investigations

Obvious gynaecological or non-gynaecological disease should be managed appropriately. Often the diagnosis is unclear and the only investigation of value in the absence of clinical findings is a laparoscopy. Fifty per cent of women with chronic pelvic pain and a normal pelvic examination will have laparoscopic abnormalities but, conversely, only 15% of women with an abnormal pelvic examination will not have an abnormality on laparoscopy.

Treatment

The treatment of any chronic pain disorder begins in the history taking with the establishment of rapport between the woman and her examining doctor. In 30% of women with chronic pain, no abnormality can be detected and the pain is therefore 'psychosomatic'. Treatment should combine support, an attempt to increase the woman's awareness of how her pain is affected by stress or emotions, and analgesia. Initially aspirin or paracetamol should be used or a prostaglandin synthetase inhibitor if dysmenorrhea is a component. Once a physical abnormality has been excluded (by physical examination and laparoscopy) the therapeutic approach can shift to the perspective of how the woman is going to deal with the pain and still function in her normal life. Trained psychological support may also be beneficial when the woman has accepted that no physical cause can be found.

Many of these women have been demonstrated to have abnormal pelvic venograms. Whether this venodilatation is a cause of, or an association with, pelvic pain is unproven. Research into this phenomenon continues in subspecialty clinics which also provide a well-organized and effective psychological support service.

Follow-up

Women with pelvic pain need to be followed for 1–2 years as a large proportion will have recurrent pain. This is a difficult management problem, particularly in those women who have had surgery for their pelvic pain (often including abdominal hysterectomy ± bilateral salpingo-oophorectomy). The corollary to this is that surgery should be avoided in the absence of obvious pathology.

10. Infertility

M. Chapman

Expectations of the examiners

The candidate will be expected to have an organized approach to the investigation and management of the infertile couple. A basic understanding of reproductive endocrinology is necessary but the more complex aspects including detailed knowledge of sophisticated drug regimens are not essential.

Definition

Infertility can be defined as the failure to conceive after a period of 12 months of unprotected intercourse. The time period is arbitrary but relates to natural rates of conception, i.e. 80% of couples will be pregnant after 12 cycles.

During the second year of attempted conception 50% of those remaining will conceive spontaneously. Subsequently the chances of conception are in the order of 50% in the following four years. Any treatment for infertility must improve that background rate of conception.

The differentiation of infertility into primary (no previous pregnancies) and secondary (previous pregnancies) is only useful in that the incidence of causes for each are different, e.g. secondary infertility is more likely to be due to tubal damage. Male factors are more likely in primary infertility.

Pathophysiology

The three major causes of infertility are:

1. Semen quality—30%
2. Ovulatory disorders—30%
3. Tubal problems—30%.

Other causes include:

1. In the male
   a. Impotence
   b. Retrograde ejaculation
   c. Antisperm antibodies

2. In the female
   a. Cervical factor (including antisperm antibodies)
   b. Endometriosis.

The diagnosis of unexplained infertility is reached after exclusion of the above causes.

Assessment

A detailed history from both partners can suggest the underlying problem(s). An assessment of the couple's general health and of their current life stresses, e.g. occupation, family problems etc., is useful to provide a background to the problem. Regularity of sexual intercourse and timing and any associated problems need to be explored with both partners. Infertility itself may contribute substantial psychological pressure and impair the ability to conceive.

Male

In the male, causes for poor semen quality should be sought.

1. Infections, e.g. mumps as an adult; gonococcal infection leading to blocked vasa deferentia
2. Operations, e.g. inguinal herniorrhaphy; orchidopexy
3. Drugs, e.g. antimitotic agents; β blockers; alcohol (in excess); nicotine.

Information about previous pregnancies should be obtained from each partner separately. Examination should be performed to assess that the genitalia are normal. The size and consistency of the testicles should be noted as well as the presence of vasa deferentia and varicocoele.

Female

In the female the history is aimed at providing evidence of ovulation. Signs and symptoms suggesting ovulation include:

1. Regular cycles
2. Mid-cycle pain (mittelschmerz)
3. Changes in vaginal discharge
4. Premenstrual symptoms, e.g. breast tenderness
5. Primary spasmodic dysmenorrhoea.

The reproductive history should be documented in detail. Factors suggesting tubal disease should be sought, i.e. pelvic inflammatory disease, previous pelvic or abdominal surgery, intrauterine device usage, chronic lower abdominal pain and secondary dysmenorrhoea. Full physical assessment including pelvic examination should be performed.

Investigations

Male

Semen analysis. Instruction for collection should include three days abstinence from ejaculation and rapid transport to the laboratory (< 1 hour) of a specimen obtained by masturbation.

Normal parameters

1. Volume: 2–5 ml
2. Concentration: > 20 million/ml
3. Motility: > 50%
4. Normal forms: > 50%.

Specimens with subnormal parameters should be repeated in 4–6 weeks before final assessment of quality is made.

Diagnostic categories

1. Normal (as above)
2. Azoospermia (no spermatozoa seen)
3. Oligospermia (concentration < 20 million/ml)
   a. Severe
   b. Moderate
   c. Mild.
4. Asthenospermia (decreased motility).

Further investigations: LH, FSH, testosterone.

Impaired semen quality is predominantly due to spermatogenic failure of unknown cause. The importance of varicocoeles in male subfertility is controversial.

Postcoital test. This test involves aspiration of a sample of cervical mucus around the time of ovulation within six hours of intercourse. A positive test, i.e. motile sperm in the cervical mucus excludes a cervical problem and confirms vaginal intercourse has occurred. A negative test can be caused by many factors other than mucus hostility e.g. poor timing and infection, and therefore its value is limited.

Female

Ovulation

Temperature charts. The basal body temperature chart has a minimal role but is worth recording for a maximum of two cycles to:

1. Define cycle length
2. Determine frequency of intercourse
3. Check biphasic pattern indicating ovulation (correlation with bio-chemical parameters of ovulation: 70–80%).

Serum progesterone. This is taken seven days prior to the menses, e.g. day 21 of 28-day cycle or day 25 of 32-day cycle. Serial measurements should be taken if the cycle is irregular. Values greater than 30 nmol/l indicate ovulation.

Other methods of assessment. These include ultrasound monitoring, direct visualization of a corpus luteum at laparoscopy, and monitoring of serum LH levels to time ovulation.

Tubal patency

Hysterosalpingogram (HSG). HSG demonstrates intrauterine and tubal anatomy and patency but it provides no information about problems elsewhere in the pelvis, e.g. adhesions. It is an outpatient procedure but generally causes discomfort or pain. There is a small risk of introducing or reactivating infection.

Laparoscopy and dye instillation. This procedure demonstrates pelvic anatomy and pathology, e.g. adhesions, endometriosis, ovarian disease and tubal patency. It is an inpatient procedure requiring general anaesthesia with an operative mortality of 1:16000. The correlation of HSG and laparoscopy findings is 70–80% and therefore it may be necessary to perform both investigations. Most women have a laparoscopy and dye instillation initially followed by an HSG if indicated.

Rubella status. This should be checked prior to commencing treatment. Non-immune patients must be vaccinated and advised to avoid pregnancy for three months.

Treatment

Male

The outlook is poor if there is azoospermia or severe oligospermia and there is no proven therapeutic approach. Cold showers, loose underwear, varicocoele ligation and hormonal strategies (except in hypopituitarism) have not been shown to be of any benefit. Mild and moderate oligospermia may improve spontaneously and pregnancies do occur. Semen preparation can significantly improve the chances of conception if GIFT (gamete intra fallopian transfer) or IVF (in vitro fertilization) are employed. Artificial insemination with donor semen is successful in 50–60% of cases (for 12 cycles) but is only acceptable to 60% of suitable couples.

Female

Ovulatory problems (see amenorrhoea). The use of ovulation induction techniques has substantially improved the chances of conception to almost normal rates. The first line of treatment is clomiphene citrate, initially 50 mg from day 2 to 6 of the menstrual cycle. Clomiphene increases FSH production by acting as an anti-oestrogen at the pituitary level. Serum progesterone levels should be checked to confirm ovulation. The use of other ovulation induction agents (gonadotrophins, LHRH analogues) are only appropriate in specialist units. The complications of ovulation induction agents include hyperstimulation and multiple pregnancy.

Tubal problems. The overall success rate of tubal surgery is 20–30%. In specialized centres, success rates in selected cases can be up to 50%.

In vitro fertilization. IVF produces a 'take home baby' rate of 15–20%. In vitro fertilization is used in cases of infertility due to tubal disease. It involves the induction of ovulation and collection of multiple ova (either by laparoscope or ultrasound guided needle aspiration) followed by extracorporeal fertilization. Embryos are replaced into the uterine cavity transcervically after 48 hours.

Unexplained infertility. This is an increasing problem and GIFT is the only treatment that has contributed significantly to successful management. GIFT involves ovulation induction and ova collection using the laparoscope. At the time of operation the ova and freshly washed semen are replaced into the fallopian tube where fertilization occurs. 'Take home baby' rates of 25–30% can be expected.

Other problems. Cervical factors and antisperm antibodies are poorly understood and difficult to treat. Spontaneous pregnancies do occur and assisted conception can be useful.

The GP's role in management

The initial investigation (except for tests of tubal patency) of an infertile couple can be performed in a general practice setting. In cases of straightforward failure of ovulation, treatment by the GP with clomiphene for 3 to 6 months is appropriate. Failure to conceive within this period necessitates specialist referral.

SUMMARY

Infertility is a common problem affecting 1:6 couples wishing to conceive. History is important and investigation should be structured to produce a diagnosis in a short time. Referral to specialist centres is mandatory if pregnancy is not achieved relatively quickly as the psychological effects of infertility can aggravate the problem.

11. Congenital abnormalities of the female genital tract

J. Rymer

Expectations of the examiners

A detailed knowledge of the abnormalities is not required but the candidate is expected to know the complications that they may produce.

Definition

An anomaly of the female genital tract that is present at birth.

Interesting facts

Women with congenital abnormalities of the uterus often have renal tract anomalies. The cause of congenital abnormalities of the genital tract is thought to be of polygenic aetiology rather than a single genetic cause.

Pathophysiology

The paramesonephric ducts (Mullerian) are the precursors of the fallopian tubes, uterus, and upper two-thirds of the vagina. The lower third of the vagina develops from the urogenital sinus. The paramesonephric ducts develop parallel to the mesonephric ducts from an invagination of coelomic epithelium. They progress caudally and cross the mesonephric ducts ventrally, and fuse to form a Y-shaped uterovaginal primordium which projects into the urogenital sinus. Canalization of the paramesonephric ducts begins before fusion of the ducts and proceeds craniocaudally. The vaginal septum disappears before the uterine septum. The uterine fundus then bulges cranially to form a convex dome.

The classification of the congenital uterine anomalies may be based on the embryological developmental defect.

1. Failure of development, e.g. no paramesonephric duct development or unilateral development
2. Failure of paramesonephric duct canalization
3. Failure of fusion of paramesonephric ducts
4. Failure of median septum loss

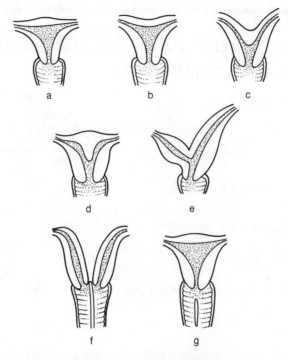

Fig. 11.1   Congenital abnormalities of the uterus and vagina.
a. Normal uterus and vagina; b. arcuate uterus; c. bicornuate uterus; d. subseptate uterus; e. rudimentary horn; f. uterus didelphys; g. normal uterus with partial vaginal septum.

5. Failure of fundal dome development
6. Failure of fusion of paramesonephric ducts with urogenital sinus
7. Failure of transverse septum loss between paramesonephric system and urogenital sinus.

See Figure 11.1.

Assessment

The following features are associated with congenital abnormalities of the uterus:

1. Primary amenorrhoea (cryptomenorrhoea)
2. Recurrent first trimester abortions
3. Recurrent second trimester abortions
4. Preterm labour
5. Abnormal fetal presentations in late pregnancy
6. Intrauterine growth retardation
7. Incoordinate uterine action
8. Retained placenta.

As many of the above features can occur with other conditions, diagnosis is difficult. A high index of suspicion is needed and diagnostic procedures should be undertaken early.

Investigations

1. Examination under anaesthesia
   a. Probing the fundus of the uterus: this may detect an arcuate uterus
   b. Passing a dilator through the cervix: if a size 7 hegar dilator can be passed through easily then cervical incompetence may be present
   c. Dilatation and curettage: this procedure should detect partial septums or double systems
2. Manual removal of the placenta
3. Hysterography: dye is injected through the cervix and X-ray pictures are taken. The uterine cavity and tubal lumens can be seen
4. Hysteroscopy
5. Ultrasound
6. Laparoscopy ± dye insufflation.

Management

Each case must be dealt with individually and depends on:

1. Time of diagnosis
2. Previous obstetric history
3. Nature of the lesion
4. Mode of presentation.

Non-pregnant

1. Cervical incompetence: this condition usually occurs after previous dilatation of the cervix, however congenital cervical incompetence can occur. A cervical cerclage can be inserted prior to pregnancy, but most are performed at 14–16 weeks of pregnancy.
2. Uteroplasty: the septum is surgically excised at laparotomy. Most operations reduce the size of the uterine cavity but the fundal dome is increased and all patients must have caesarean sections in subsequent pregnancies.
3. Hysteroscopic incision of the uterine septum: under direct visualization through a hysteroscope the uterine septa is divided, either surgically or by laser. The uterus remains arcuate.

During pregnancy

1. Cervical cerclage: ideally performed at 14–16 weeks. The suture is

removed at about 37 weeks. If the woman goes into spontaneous labour prior to this the suture must be removed.
2. Bedrest: the benefit has not been ascertained.
3. Intrauterine growth retardation: placentation on the septum may cause IUGR and patients must be managed appropriately.

During labour

1. Incoordinate uterine action: if inefficient uterine action results because of congenital abnormality of the uterus this should be corrected with oxytocin.
2. Malpresentations or fetal distress are dealt with appropriately.
3. Vaginal septum: this can be excised if there is delayed progress in the second stage of labour.
4. Retained placenta: as the incidence of retained placenta is increased, active management of the third stage is required (see Ch. 25).

SUMMARY

As it is so difficult to diagnose congenital abnormalities of the uterus, it is difficult to assess the various forms of treatment. In cases of recurrent first trimester abortions, midtrimester abortions, preterm labour, and retained placentae, the index of suspicion should be high.

12. Hirsutism and virilism

M. Chapman

Expectations of the examiners

Hirsutism is a common complaint which is not usually managed particularly well. The examiners will expect a limited understanding of the physiology of androgen metabolism. Candidates should have a knowledge of basic investigations, their interpretation and subsequent management. Specialist endocrinological referral will be part of the management in severe cases.

Definition

Hirsutism can be defined as excessive hair growth outside the normal female distribution. Difficulties have arisen in defining 'normal' from 'abnormal'.

Virilism is defined as masculinization of the female involving one or more of the following features: clitoral hypertrophy, muscle hypertrophy, breast atrophy, hirsutism, deepening of the voice.

Interesting facts

Hirsutism is common. Depending on the stringency of the definition, more than 10% of females could be deemed to be hirsute. Only a small proportion complain.

Management of the psychological effects of hirsutism is the most important aspect of this problem. In almost all cases the underlying hormonal imbalance is benign.

Virilism is extremely rare (< 1% patients referred with hirsutism).

Pathophysiology

The physiology of the androgens is complex. There are many androgens with differing relative biological activities which are produced from a variety of sites. For example, dehydroepiandrosterone (DHEA), is produced predominantly by the adrenal gland and has a very weak biological activity when compared to testosterone. Dihydrotestosterone

(DHT), which has greater biological activity, is produced by peripheral conversion of weaker androgens.

Binding of the androgens to sex hormone binding globulin (SHBG) and albumin reduces the availability of the free steroid.

In hirsutism, various disorders of androgen metabolism can occur. Production rates of the androgens can be increased from the ovary (e.g. in polycystic ovarian disease) or the adrenal gland (e.g. in the case of a tumour) or peripheral conversion can be enhanced (e.g. in obesity or increased precursor production). SHBG may be reduced in liver disease. Finally, there may be an increased sensitivity of target organs to normal levels of testosterone (e.g. hair follicles, clitoris).

Aetiology

1. Ovarian
   a. Polycystic ovarian disease
   b. Tumour, e.g. androblastomas, teratomas
2. Adrenal
   a. Androgen secreting tumours
   b. Cushing's syndrome
   c. Congenital adrenal hyperplasia
3. Idiopathic
4. Rare causes
   a. Drugs
   b. Familial hypertrichosis
   c. Virilized intersexual disorders.

Assessment

Specific points in the history include:

Menstrual pattern

A regular menstrual cycle excludes a significant underlying hormonal disturbance. Oligo- or amenorrhoea should be investigated fully to look for polycystic ovarian syndrome and to exclude the rarer but potentially life-threatening hormone-secreting tumours.

Racial group and family history

Hair distribution varies substantially with racial group, e.g. Scandinavian women rarely have facial hair whereas in South Mediterranean women it is common.

Drugs

E.g. Danazol, testosterone implant.

Examination should exclude endocrine disease and signs of virilism should be noted. The severity of the hirsutism should be assessed and specific enquiry should be made about previous local treatments.

Investigations

Plasma androgens

A normal or slightly elevated testosterone level suggests a benign cause for the hirsutism. High levels are strongly suggestive of an androgen-secreting tumour. Raised serum DHEA and androstenedione levels indicate an adrenal origin of the excess androgens. Raised levels of 17-hydroxy-progesterone may indicate congenital adrenal hyperplasia.

SHBG

SHBG binds testosterone and reduces the free testosterone available to stimulate receptors in the hair follicles. A low level of SHBG is associated with a raised total testosterone level and a higher concentration of free testosterone.

Gonadotrophin levels

Raised LH levels and increased LH/FSH ratios are consistent with poly-cystic ovarian disease.

Other

Further investigations of specific endocrine disorders should be performed as indicated.

Treatment

Serious conditions should be excluded.

Psychological

The benign nature of the condition should be explained and continuing support may be necessary.

Local treatment

This may be the most effective management and includes:

1. Bleaching agents
2. Plucking
3. Shaving
4. Depilatory creams
5. Waxes
6. Electrolysis: this is effective and permanent but it can be painful and occasionally leave scarring.

Drugs

1. Dexamethasone: adrenal (ovarian) suppression
2. Oral contraceptives: SHBG elevation
3. Cyproterone acetate
4. Spironolactone: androgen receptor inhibition.

In general practice it is appropriate to use dexamethasone or oral contraceptives but further drug therapy should be prescribed after specialist referral.

It is important to emphasize that the pharmacological therapy of hirsutism is lengthy (12 to 24 months). Immediate improvement should not be expected.

SUMMARY

A detailed history and examination usually provides the diagnosis but basic investigations will confirm the presence of benign androgen excess. Reassurance can then be provided and advice about cosmetic treatment should be given. More severe cases should be managed by a gynaecologist or an endocrinologist.

13. Bleeding in early pregnancy

G. Davis

Expectations of the examiners

Bleeding in early pregnancy is common and candidates will be expected to differentiate between those patients who can be managed at home and those requiring admission, and to have a knowledge of the clinical findings which distinguish the two groups. In terms of clinical management, the important diagnostic decision is between threatened abortion and the remainder, but the terminology encourages examiners to ask about definitions.

Definitions

Abortion. Termination of pregnancy prior to 28 weeks' gestation, either spontaneous or induced.

Threatened abortion. Bleeding in early pregnancy without dilatation of the cervix or the passage of products of conception (POC).

Inevitable abortion. Bleeding in early pregnancy associated with cervical dilatation but without passage of POC.

Incomplete abortion. Bleeding in early pregnancy with cervical dilatation and the passage of POC.

Complete abortion. Bleeding in early pregnancy followed by the passage of all POC.

Missed abortion. Early pregnancy in which the fetus dies and the uterus fails to enlarge further. There may or may not be bleeding.

Septic abortion. Any abortion that becomes infected.

SPONTANEOUS ABORTION

Interesting facts

The commonly quoted incidence for abortion is 15%, but is probably much higher (40–60%) when early pregnancies are included, i.e. prior to detection. These biochemical pregnancies probably present as slightly delayed periods which may be heavier than normal. Most spontaneous abortions occur prior to 12 weeks' gestation with a peak incidence at 7–8 weeks. The frequency of abortion increases with maternal age, smoking and alcohol consumption.

Aetiology

1. Fetal abnormalities. These account for more than 50% of all spontaneous abortions and include chromosomal and developmental abnormalities. Chromosomal abnormalities (most commonly trisomy) are present in 80% of pregnancies in which a conceptus is not present (otherwise known as a blighted embryo or an afetal sac).
2. Uterine abnormalities. Malformation of the uterus may interfere with normal development of the pregnancy. Abnormalities may be congenital or acquired, e.g. submucous fibroids or mechanical damage from previous curettage.
3. Systemic disease. Most severe systemic diseases, e.g. connective tissue and renal disease, increase the rate of abortion. Any systemic infection or sustained pyrexia may cause abortion. Infections are not a common cause, but cytomegalovirus, toxoplasmosis and rubella are classically associated with an increased risk of abortion. Similarly, listeriosis and syphilis are uncommon causes of abortion in the second trimester.
4. Drugs. Cytotoxic drugs, particularly antimetabolites, will cause abortion.
5. Immunological. There has been considerable debate on this subject and it has more relevance to, and is briefly reviewed in, the following section on recurrent abortion.
6. Vascular. An abnormal uterine arterial blood supply is associated with an increased risk of spontaneous abortion, possibly as a result of inadequate blood flow to the developing placenta.
7. Psychological. There is no convincing evidence that stress alone can cause abortion.

Assessment

History

1. Period of amenorrhoea.
2. Amount of bleeding.
3. Degree of pain.
4. Time of onset of pain in relation to bleeding (i.e. if the pain started first, ectopic pregnancy is more likely).
5. Whether products have been passed. This is very unreliable as organized clot is difficult to distinguish from products of conception.

Examination

There are five clinical findings of relevance:

1. The cardiovascular status of the patient.
2. Abdominal palpation. The uterus or lower abdomen may be tender,

there should be no rebound tenderness and the pain is not usually unilateral. The exception is septic abortion where the whole of the lower abdomen may be tender with guarding and rebound. The diagnosis is usually obvious as the woman is febrile, toxic, and abdominal tenderness is marked.
3. State of the cervix—whether it is starting to dilate.
4. Whether any products are visible.
5. Uterine size should be equivalent to the expected size for the period of amenorrhoea.

Investigations

1. Ultrasound scan (USS). In the absence of confirmed POC or cervical dilatation a USS is the definitive investigation in the management of abortion. If an intrauterine pregnancy is present, 45% will abort spontaneously, however, if viability is confirmed by ultrasound 95–98% of these women will progress to a normal outcome in that pregnancy. Ultrasound can reliably detect a live intrauterine pregnancy after six weeks' gestation.
2. FBC. To assess blood loss and serve as a baseline.
3. Blood group and save. If bleeding is significant, blood may need to be crossmatched and transfused. Rhesus status must be known prior to discharge from hospital and the appropriate action taken.
4. Septic abortions will require blood cultures and endocervical swabs. Further investigations will be required if the woman is septicaemic.

Treatment

Threatened abortion

The conventional management is bed rest and abstinence from intercourse. Progesterone supplementation has also been used. There is no evidence that any of these measures affect the outcome of the pregnancy. Hospital admission is not necessary but may be appropriate in selected cases.

Incomplete, inevitable, missed abortion

All require admission to hospital and evacuation of the uterus. Any products visible in the os at the initial examination should be removed with a pair of sponge-holding forceps. Failure to do so can allow the patient to go into 'cervical shock', i.e. cardiogenic shock thought to be related to vagal stimulation as a result of cervical dilatation. Ergometrine, 0.5 mg i.m. may be useful in reducing blood loss and raising the blood pressure.

Septic abortion

The treatment of septic abortion is based on the principles of resuscitation, adequate antibiotic coverage and evacuation of the uterus when the patient's condition permits. In practice this usually means 12–24 hours of preoperative intravenous antibiotics, a broad-spectrum agent (such as a cephalosporin) and metronidazole, and gentamicin if the patient is septicaemic.

Evacuation of the uterus

This is usually performed with suction and completed with gentle curettage to ensure the uterus is empty. Particular care is necessary in septic abortion because of the increased risk of perforation.

Complications

1. Immediate
   a. Haemorrhage
   b. Infection
   c. Uterine perforation
2. Delayed
   a. Infertility
   b. Asherman's syndrome—complete or partial loss of the endometrium due to excessive curettage
   c. Cervical incompetence—whether this occurs after spontaneous abortion is debatable.

Follow-up

Anti-D γ-globulin should be given to rhesus-negative women. Suppression of lactation is not usually necessary before 20 weeks. Prior to discharge the causes and prognosis should be discussed with the woman (and partner if possible). After abortion in the first pregnancy the chance of abortion in the next pregnancy is about 15–20% and slightly higher, 25–30%, after the first two pregnancies abort. The emotional reaction to abortion is variable and some women require full bereavement counselling. The Miscarriage Association is a patient-organized support group which many women find helpful (see Appendix for address). Avoidance of pregnancy for at least six and preferably 12 months may be recommended for psychological reasons but each couple must be dealt with on an individual basis.

RECURRENT ABORTION

Definition

Loss of three consecutive pregnancies of less than 28 weeks' gestation.

Interesting facts

The incidence of recurrent abortion is widely quoted as being 1% of the child-bearing population. The mean gestational age of recurrent abortions tends to be greater than sporadic abortions. If the couple already have a live child the incidence of three subsequent consecutive abortions is halved. Overall, the likelihood of a successful pregnancy following three previous abortions is about 60–75%.

Aetiology

Chromosome abnormalities

Although this is an important cause, they are more common in sporadic than repeated abortions. Couples who recurrently abort have an increased incidence (4%) of chromosomal abnormalities but usually different abnormalities to those found in the conceptus, i.e. there may be a familial susceptibility to chromosomal rearrangement.

Uterine abnormalities

Cervical incompetence

The diagnosis of cervical incompetence is a retrospective one based on a history of mid-trimester abortion associated with painless cervical dilatation or rupture of the membranes. It is almost certainly over-diagnosed and overtreated. There is often, but not invariably, a history of previous surgical dilatation of the cervix or cervical surgery such as cone biopsy. True cervical incompetence causes recurrent abortion and is treated surgically by the insertion of a cervical suture at 12–14 weeks gestation. The Shirodkar suture has now been replaced by the technically simpler McDonald suture which is inserted under general anaesthesia and removed at 36–38 weeks' gestation.

Immunology

In normal pregnancy the genetic dissimilarity between the parents in some unknown way triggers production of a 'blocking factor(s)' which prevents maternal lymphocytes from reacting to, and destroying, fetal cells. It has been suggested that with couples in whom recurrent abortions occur there are immunological similarities and, as a result, a blocking factor is not produced. This hypothesis has led to extensive research and the empirical treatment of women who recurrently abort with transfusion of either donor whole blood or their partner's lymphocytes to try and stimulate the production of blocking factor. Rates for subsequent successful pregnancy are 75–80% but it must be remembered that the expected rate of successful pregnancy after three consecutive abortions is 60–75% and a success rate of

86% has been reported after treatment with psychological support alone. At present, the relationship between unexplained recurrent abortion and the immunological status of the parents has still to be determined.

Hormonal abnormalities

Some women who recurrently abort have lower levels of progesterone in the luteal phase and in early pregnancy. However, progesterone therapy does not improve fetal survival, suggesting that the low progesterone levels are a result of impaired placental development rather than a cause.

Systemic disease

The evidence that thyroid disease or diabetes cause recurrent (or sporadic) abortions is unconvincing. However, other systemic diseases do cause abortion and of particular interest in this regard is recurrent second trimester abortion associated with the presence of the lupus anticoagulant (which paradoxically causes thrombosis). Even in the presence of other signs of connective tissue disease, if circulating levels of anticoagulant can be suppressed by steroids then a good outcome can be achieved. The importance of this is that it is one of the few treatable causes of abortion.

Assessment

1. History of pregnancy loss
    a. How many?
    b. What gestation?
    c. Was there pain or bleeding?
    d. Were they all with one partner?
2. Medical history
    a. Previous cervical dilatation
    b. Previous curettage
    c. Previous sexually transmitted disease
    d. Systemic disease.
3. Family history of recurrent abortion.
4. Examination is usually not helpful but should include general physical and pelvic examination.

Investigations

1. Most important
    a. Chromosome analysis of couple
    b. Hysterosalpingogram
2. Less important
    a. FBC

   b. Urea, creatinine, MSU (renal disease)
   c. Serological tests for syphilis
   d. Rubella
   e. Hepatitis B.

Treatment

Immunotherapy has been briefly discussed. Most couples simply need emotional support and information. The important fact is that 60–75% will have a normal pregnancy after three consecutive spontaneous abortions. A major contribution of recurrent abortion clinics (most of which have been set up to provide immunotherapy) has been in providing support for these couples. A few specific abnormalities can be treated: intrauterine adhesions can be broken down surgically by using a hysteroscope and an intrauterine device inserted for three to six months to prevent adhesions reforming. The successful pregnancy rate has been reported to increase after this. The role of myomectomy in improving outcome is debated. The use of cervical cerclage has been discussed.

THERAPEUTIC ABORTION

Definition

Medical termination of pregnancy prior to 24 weeks' gestation. The implications of the 1990 modifications are unknown at this time.

Features

Since the 1967 Abortion Act, termination of pregnancy is possible in England and Wales providing it is carried out by a registered medical practitioner and two registered medical practitioners have signed the appropriate consent form (Certificate A) in a licensed place. The grounds for abortion under the Act are:

1. The continuance of the pregnancy would involve risk to the life of the pregnant woman greater than if the pregnancy were terminated.
2. The continuance of the pregnancy would involve risk of injury to physical or mental health of the pregnant woman greater than if the pregnancy were terminated.
3. The continuance of the pregnancy would involve risk of injury to the physical or mental health of the existing child(ren) of the pregnant woman greater than if the pregnancy were terminated.
4. There is substantial risk that if the child were born it would suffer from such physical or mental abnormalities as to be seriously handicapped.

    The vast majority of therapeutic abortions are carried out on the basis of the second reason—risk to the physical or mental health of the woman. In

1982–1984, abortions comprised 17% of total births and abortions, i.e. about one in six pregnancies were terminated.

The rate of legal terminations has remained static in the 1980s, except in 1988 when there was an 8% increase for unknown reasons. Most NHS hospitals provide a termination service and there are a number of private clinics and private gynaecologists who also provide this service.

Assessment

Assuming that the practitioner follows the woman's (and partner's, if present) wishes, three pieces of information are required:

1. Is she pregnant and, if so, what is the gestation?
2. Does the woman definitely want an abortion?
3. Is she fit for an anaesthetic?

Abortion services should provide counselling so that the woman's commitment can be adequately assessed and she can have the opportunity to discuss her decision in a supportive environment. As most women are referred by their general practitioner, they should have discussed it with him/her and the doctor should sign the medical consent form which the woman can bring with her.

History

1. Pregnancy
   a. Period of amenorrhoea
   b. Menstrual cycle
   c. Previous contraception
   d. Symptoms of pregnancy
2. Past medical and obstetric history.

Examination

1. Physical examination
2. Uterine size.

Investigations

1. Ultrasound scan if > 14 weeks' gestation to confirm gestation
2. FBC
3. Group and save.

Methods

Most terminations of pregnancy in England and Wales are carried out under general anaesthesia but in other countries local anaesthesia is used up to 12 weeks' gestation. This has the advantage of avoiding the risks of general anaesthesia and reducing blood loss, but requires greater involvement by both staff and patients.

Prior to 12 weeks:

Suction aspiration. Used routinely up to 12 weeks' gestation. The cervix is dilated and a semirigid plastic suction catheter is inserted into the uterus. Most operators check that evacuation is complete with sponge forceps and *gentle* curettage.

RU486. The new progesterone antagonist, RU486, in association with a prostaglandin pessary is 99% effective in termination of pregnancy prior to 8 weeks' gestation without recourse to operation. Provided that anti-abortion opinion allows its general introduction, it represents the biggest single advance in the field since the 1967 Act. *Approved. 63 days.*

After 12 weeks:

Dilatation and evacuation. After 12 weeks' gestation, instrumental destruction and removal of the pieces is employed, often in conjunction with suction aspiration to reduce the uterine volume. A bolus of 5–10 U of syntocinon is often given intravenously during or after the procedure. This method is commonly used up to 16 weeks' gestation and by a few operators up to 20–22 weeks.

Prostaglandins (PG) are used for second trimester terminations, usually after 16 weeks. They may be administered as repeated, frequent vaginal pessaries, infusion extra-amniotically into the uterine cavity, or (most commonly) as an intra-amniotic bolus injection. PG by any route, but particularly if inadvertently given intravenously, may cause systemic side-effects of nausea, vomiting, sweating, bronchospasm or diarrhoea. Usually these symptoms are not prominent but resuscitation equipment and adrenaline must be readily available.

PG are used for most late terminations but the terminations may be prolonged (12–48 hours) and require considerable analgesia. Often a syntocinon infusion is added to accelerate the onset of labour (despite the relative insensitivity of the uterus to oxytocin until the third trimester).

Hysterotomy is very rarely used in modern practice. The major reason for avoiding its use is the risk of rupture of the uterine scar in subsequent pregnancy.

Complications

The risk of complications is directly related to the experience of the operator and the gestation of the pregnancy.

1. Immediate
   a. General anaesthesia
   b. Uterine perforation—usually this is not major and the woman can be

observed, but any evidence of continuing bleeding necessitates laparotomy and closure of the uterine defect
c. Incomplete evacuation leading to haemorrhage or infection.
2. Delayed
a. Infertility due to postoperative infection
b. Asherman's syndrome (see above)
c. Cervical incompetence (see above)
d. Psychological—the response is very variable but can be prolonged and significant. Future subfertility is often correctly and incorrectly attributed to previous termination of pregnancy.

Follow-up

In practice, very few centres follow up their patients despite the frequency of emotional difficulties most women experience after termination of pregnancy.

EXTRAUTERINE PREGNANCY

Definition

Implantation of a pregnancy outside the uterine cavity, the majority in the fallopian tube (95%).

Interesting facts

In the 1982–1984 Maternal Mortality report for England and Wales, ectopic pregnancy was the sixth commonest cause of maternal mortality (10 cases). The initial diagnosis is incorrect in 25–50% of cases. Its incidence (one in 200 pregnancies) has doubled in the past 20 years and varies in different groups, e.g. one in 30 pregnancies in the West Indies and in 2–3% of pregnancies resulting from assisted conception.

The diagnosis is usually made late and delay between admission and operation is common. The classic symptoms of ectopic pregnancy are abdominal pain, amenorrhoea, and irregular vaginal bleeding. The diagnostic problem is that these symptoms are also associated with spontaneous abortion and pelvic inflammatory disease, the two commonest alternative diagnoses. Shock is present in 15–25% of cases. It is unclear how many would or do resolve spontaneously.

Predisposing factors

Pelvic inflammatory disease (PID). Histological evidence for previous pelvic infection can be found in 30–50% of ectopic gestations. Evidence suggests that previous infection increases the risk of ectopic pregnancy about 10 times. It is widely believed that the recent increase in ectopic pregnancy is related to the current epidemic in PID.

Tubal surgery. Any form of surgery to the tubes including sterilization increases the ratio of ectopic to intrauterine pregnancy.

Previous tubal pregnancy. The risk of subsequent pregnancy implanting ectopically is increased 20-fold even if salpingectomy has been performed. This is presumably because the predisposing pathology (i.e. tubal damage) is bilateral.

Infertility. Pregnancy in subfertile women, whether after induction of ovulation or assisted conception techniques (IVF or GIFT) is more likely to implant ectopically. In many cases this is due to pre-existing tubal disease.

Intrauterine devices. The overall incidence of ectopic pregnancy in IUD users is lower than normal. However, if pregnancy occurs, the ratio of ectopic to intrauterine pregnancies is one in 20.

Progestins. The low dose progestagen-only pills have a similar effect to IUDs in that they increase the ectopic to intrauterine pregnancy ratio while not affecting, or slightly reducing, the overall incidence of ectopic pregnancy. However, the addition of progestin to an inert IUD (Progestasert) appears to increase the incidence of ectopic pregnancy three-fold over non-contraceptive users. The reasons for this are unclear.

Assessment

The most important aid to diagnosis is a high level of suspicion—all women in the reproductive age group who present with one or any combination of the symptoms i.e. abdominal pain, vaginal bleeding and amenorrhoea, should be assumed to have an ectopic pregnancy until proven otherwise.

History

1. Pain
   a. *Usually* unilateral but may be bilateral
   b. Usually starts prior to the bleeding
   c. May radiate to the shoulder tip
2. Bleeding
   a. Classically dark red and described as 'prune juice'
   b. Usually not as heavy as in spontaneous abortion
   c. May pass a decidual cast, mimicking products of conception
3. Amenorrhoea: *Absent* in 25% of cases.

Examination

1. Cardiovascular status—may be shocked

2. Abdomen—unilateral tenderness usually with rebound but may present with a rigid abdomen if massive blood loss
3. Uterus enlarged, cervical excitation is usually present and a mass may be palpable although in half of these the ectopic pregnancy will be on the opposite side.

Investigations

In the collapsed, shocked patient, no investigations are required prior to surgery. In less obvious cases the following investigations are necessary.

Pregnancy test. Sensitive tests for B-HCG will be positive in $> 95\%$ of ectopic pregnancies although less sensitive tests are less reliable.

Ultrasound scan. If an intrauterine pregnancy is detected the diagnosis of ectopic pregnancy can virtually be excluded. The coexistence of intra-uterine and ectopic pregnancies is rare (1 in 30 000) except in assisted conception. The problem arises in pregnancies at four to six weeks' gestation where the sac is not visible. These patients require laparoscopy.

Laparoscopy. All women who present with pain and bleeding, a positive pregnancy test or B-HCG and no intrauterine pregnancy on ultrasound should have an urgent laparoscopy. Undiagnosed unilateral pain (without a positive pregnancy test) which does not resolve within 24–48 hours should also be investigated by laparoscopy to exclude ectopic pregnancy.

Other investigations.

1. FBC
2. Cross match.

Treatment

Resuscitation. An i.v. line and resuscitation should be initiated, en route to theatre in severe cases.

Surgery. Every attempt should be made to conserve the tube. The operation of choice is controversial, ranging from salpingectomy to linear salpingotomy—opening the tube lengthwise along its antimesenteric border over the implantation site. There is no evidence that removal of the ovary on the same side affects the prognosis for future fertility in any way.

Surgery for extratubal pregnancies (e.g. ovarian or intra-abdominal pregnancies) should achieve a balance between removing the pregnancy and damaging the site of implantation. Haemostasis is often a major problem.

Prognosis

1. Immediate postoperative complications are uncommon. Occasionally if the pregnancy is 'milked out' of the fimbral end, residual trophoblast

may continue to grow, requiring further surgery. Routine postoperative management and follow-up should be undertaken.

2. Future pregnancy: only one-third of women wishing to have a further pregnancy will succeed in having a child and 10% will have a further ectopic pregnancy. The chances of intrauterine pregnancy depend on the extent of tubal damage pre- and postoperatively.

3. Undiagnosed ectopic pregnancy may result in tubal abortion into the peritoneal cavity with subsequent reabsorption of the products or rarely, abdominal implantation. Chronic bleeding from an ectopic pregnancy can lead to a pelvic haematocoele—a pelvic haematoma surrounded by inflammatory change and adhesions.

HYDATIDIFORM MOLE

Definition

A benign tumour of trophoblast.

Features

The incidence in the UK is lower (1 in 2000 pregnancies) than in South-East Asia (1 in 200 pregnancies). The aetiology is unknown and there are two types which are genetically and clinically dissimilar: complete (classical) in which no fetus is present; and partial where a fetus (or fetal material) is present. Complete moles are rare. The cells contain 46 chromosomes of *paternal* origin and they may lead to choriocarcinoma. Partial moles are more common; they have 69 chromosomes (triploid) of which the additional haploid set are again paternal in origin and probably do not give rise to choriocarcinoma. A mole may become 'invasive' and penetrate the uterus and/or metastasize, particularly to the lungs. This is distinct from choriocarcinoma which is a malignant tumour of trophoblast.

Pathology

Complete mole

There is a triad of microscopic features:

1. Hyperplasia of both syncytio- and cytotrophoblast
2. Villous oedema forming multiple small collections of fluid 'cisterns'
3. Absence of a fetus.

Partial mole

The placenta shows *focal* hyperplasia which is usually confined to the syncytiotrophoblast, and focal villous swelling with cistern formation. The fetus usually dies early and the only remnants may be the presence of erythrocytes in placental vessels. The diagnosis may be difficult as villi are often swollen in aborted tissue so the diagnosis rests with the pathologist. Where a fetus is present, multiple congenital abnormalities are evident, consistent with the triploid state.

Assessment

Moles usually present with irregular vaginal bleeding in pregnancy. The massive production of B-HCG may lead to exaggerated symptoms of pregnancy.

History

1. Amenorrhoea
2. Bleeding
3. Hyperemesis (25–30%)
4. Passage of grape-like vesicles
5. Rarely, metastatic spread: haemoptysis, pleuritic pain.

Examination

1. Pre-eclampsia may develop early (15–20%)
2. Uterus is usually larger than dates (55%), but may be smaller (15–20%)
3. Fetal heart is usually absent
4. Theca lutein cysts may be palpable (10–20%).

Investigations

1. Ultrasound: scanning reveals a typical 'snow storm' appearance in the uterus. A fetus is not usually identified
2. B-HCG is elevated, usually massively
3. Chest X-ray to exclude pulmonary metastasis.

Treatment

Suction evacuation. This may need to be repeated if bleeding persists or HCG levels are still elevated six weeks after initial evacuation. This will cure 90% of patients. The risk of perforation is increased.

Extra-amniotic prostaglandin infusion if the uterus is thought to be too large for surgical evacuation.

Hysterectomy may be performed in older women as they have a greater risk of developing choriocarcinoma.

Follow-up. All patients with molar pregnancy should be registered at a centre for trophoblastic disease. Meticulous follow-up of all women with molar pregnancies is essential. Estimations of B-HCG should be performed three weeks post-evacuation and then fortnightly until negative. They should then be assessed monthly for two years. Any rise or plateau in the B-HCG levels requires chemotherapy as outlined below under chorio-carcinoma. These cases (10%) usually become evident between three and six weeks after evacuation.

Prognosis

The mortality from trophoblastic disease is 6–8 women per year in the UK. The incidence of hydatidiform mole in a subsequent pregnancy is 1 in 120. Pregnancy is contraindicated for one year and oral contraception is not recommended. In subsequent pregnancies, women are asked to attend early for exclusion of molar pregnancy by ultrasound and a B-HCG should be performed three weeks after delivery.

CHORIOCARCINOMA

Definition

Malignant tumour of trophoblast.

Interesting facts

This may follow normal or molar pregnancy but choriocarcinoma is a thousand-fold more common after molar pregnancy, i.e. a woman presenting with choriocarcinoma has an equal chance of the preceding pregnancy being normal or molar. One in 30 moles become chorio-carcinoma and it is vastly more common in South-east Asia.

Local extension is frequent and metastatic spread is usually vascular to the lungs (70%) or brain.

Treatment

1. Methotrexate and folinic acid plus evacuation of the uterus or hysterectomy.
2. Resistant or high-risk cases require combination chemotherapy.
3. Invasive mole and choriocarcinoma are treated similarly, the treatment depending more on risk factors such as age and degree of spread than histology.
4. Follow-up of B-HCG levels is required similar to that in molar pregnancy.

Prognosis

Remission can be expected in all women except the few with metastases other than pulmonary. Pregnancy after choriocarcinoma is possible after two years free of disease and is managed in a similar way to pregnancy following other trophoblastic disease.

14. Benign conditions of the female genital tract

A. Rodin

Interesting facts

Benign lesions of the female genital tract are common and they may be congenital or acquired. Occasionally, they are manifestations of systemic disease.

THE VULVA

Abnormal appearance of the external genitalia at birth may represent an intersex state; further discussion of intersex is beyond the scope of this book. Clitoromegaly may occur in certain virilizing conditions (see Hirsutism and Virilism, Ch. 12).

PRURITUS VULVAE

Vulval irritation can occur at any age and it may be an extremely distressing symptom. It is most commonly caused by *Candida albicans* infection.

Management of this complaint is aimed at identifying the cause and then treating appropriately. A history is taken and a physical examination is

Table 14.1 Causes of pruritus vulvae.

Local causes:
   Infection
      Candida albicans
      Herpes genitalis
      Genital warts
      Other sexually transmitted diseases
      Threadworms, pubic lice, scabies
   Atrophic vulvitis
   Vulval dystrophies
   Tumours

General causes
   Skin diseases, e.g. eczema, psoriasis
   Medical conditions, e.g. diabetes mellitus, hypothyroidism, liver disease, chronic renal failure, Crohn's disease, polycythaemia
   Drug reactions
   Psychogenic

performed to look for generalized causes of pruritus. The vulva is inspected and a gentle speculum examination is performed and microbiological swabs are taken prior to digital examination. Glycosuria should be excluded and blood tests should be performed as clinically indicated. Skin biopsies should be taken if epithelial changes are suspected.

CHRONIC EPITHELIAL DYSTROPHIES OF THE VULVA

The chronic vulval dystrophies are of unknown aetiology and mainly occur in postmenopausal women. They are classified according to their histological appearance.

Classification of vulval dystrophies

1. Hyperplastic dystrophy
   a. Without atypia
   b. With atypia
2. Hypoplastic dystrophy
3. Mixed dystrophy
   a. Without atypia
   b. With atypia.

Pruritus vulvae is the commonest symptom and on examination the vulva appears atrophic and white plaques (leukoplakia) may be present. Fusion of the labia may occur with stenosis of the introitus. The changes do not extend into the vagina. The diagnosis is confirmed by histological examination of skin biopsies.

In hypoplastic dystrophy (lichen scerosis et atrophicus) there is thinning of the epidermis with hyperkeratosis and chronic inflammation in the dermis. Hyperplastic dystrophy is characterized by thickening and hyperplasia of the epidermis. Leukoplakia describes thickening and whitening of the skin and is seen in several conditions. Malignant change may occur in dystrophy associated with the presence of nuclear atypia.

Treatment

Topical

1. Corticosteroid cream   hyperplastic
2. Testosterone cream ⎫
3. Oestrogen cream.   ⎬ hypoplastic

Local

1. Laser
2. Cryosurgery.

Table 14.2   Causes of swellings of the vulva.

General causes
    Sebaceous cyst
    Haematoma
    Varicose veins
    Benign tumours, e.g. lipoma, papilloma, fibroma, hidradenoma
    Malignant tumour: primary/secondary

Specific causes
    Bartholin's gland: cyst/abscess
    Urethral caruncle
    Endometriosis
    Carcinoma of the vulva
    Inguinal hernia
    Hydrocoele of Canal of Nuck

Surgery

Vulvectomy is usually reserved for cases in which there is nuclear atypia but may be used to provide palliation in cases where there is intractable pruritus vulvae.

VULVAL LUMPS AND SWELLINGS

Lumps and swellings of the vulva are common and in the majority of cases they are benign. Any skin condition may affect the vulva.

Bartholin's gland swellings

The Bartholin's glands are paired structures which lie deep to the posterior ends of the labia minora posteriorly. The duct on each side opens between the labium minus and the hymen and is about 0.5 cm long. Normally the gland cannot be palpated. Obstruction of the duct results in accumulation of secretions and cyst formation. Women present with a painless vulval swelling. A Bartholin's abscess is painful and women present with a tender, red and sometimes fluctuant lump. Treatment of both cysts and abscesses is by marsupialization. This involves making an elliptical incision into the roof of the cyst, draining the cavity and suturing the cyst wall to the skin to allow continuing drainage. Excision of the Bartholin's gland is rarely performed.

Urethral caruncle

This term is applied to any reddened area involving the posterior margin of the urethral orifice and is thought to be due to prolapse of the posterior urethral wall. Caruncles are often symptomless and are usually found in postmenopausal women. They occasionally cause bleeding and dyspareunia. Treatment with topical oestrogen cream is usually effective but sometimes surgical excision is necessary.

Causes of vulval ulceration

See Sexually transmitted diseases (Ch. 36).

VAGINA

VAGINAL SEPTUM

See Congenital abnormalities (Ch. 11).

VAGINITIS

See Sexually transmitted diseases (Ch. 36).

VAGINAL CYSTS

These are usually remnants of the lower portion of the mesonephric (Wolffian) duct and they occur anterolaterally in the vagina. They are usually asymptomatic and require no treatment.

THE CERVIX

The vaginal portion of the cervix is covered by stratified squamous epithelium and the endocervical canal is lined by columnar epithelium. Before puberty, the squamocolumnar junction is in the endocervical canal. During adolescence, the ovarian hormones cause eversion of the lower part of the cervical canal so that columnar epithelium appears on the ectocervix. The columnar epithelium is exposed to the acid environment of the vagina and columnar epithelium is replaced by stratified squamous epithelium (squamous metaplasia). If the process of squamous metaplasia results in the obstruction of cervical glands, retention cysts may form which are known as Nabothian follicles.

CERVICAL ECTROPION

Eversion of the lower cervical canal occurs during adolescence, during pregnancy and while taking the combined oral contraceptive pill. The florid appearance of the cervix in these situations gives rise to the term 'erosion', however this is a misnomer and should be avoided.

Ectropion may also result from cervical tears sustained during childbirth. Cervical ectropion is usually asymptomatic, but occasionally causes excessive vaginal discharge or postcoital bleeding. A cervical smear should be taken. Treatment is rarely necessary but women with persistent symptoms can be treated as outpatients with cryocautery.

CERVICITIS

Chronic cervicitis is a nonspecific condition which is difficult to define. It is a common clinical diagnosis which is rarely confirmed by bacteriology.

CERVICAL POLYPS

These develop from the endocervix and protrude from the external os into the vagina. They are covered by columnar epithelium which often undergoes squamous metaplasia. They are usually asymptomatic, but the dependent part of the polyp may ulcerate causing intermenstrual and postcoital bleeding. They may also cause an increase in vaginal discharge. Cervical polyps are rarely malignant.

Cervical polyps should be avulsed and sent for histological examination. Their base should be cauterized to prevent regrowth and an endometrial biopsy should be taken at the same time to exclude other causes of irregular vaginal bleeding.

THE BODY OF THE UTERUS

POLYPS

Various types of polyps form in the cavity of the uterus including:

1. Endometrial polyps (adenomatous)
2. Fibroid polyps
3. Placental polyps.

Endometrial polyps are the most common and may be multiple in premenopausal women but are usually single in postmenopausal women. Occasionally they extrude through the cervix causing dysmenorrhoea. They may be symptomless but usually present with abnormal vaginal bleeding. Menorrhagia and intermenstrual bleeding may occur and in the older woman there may be postmenopausal bleeding. If the polyp has passed through the cervix there may be postcoital bleeding. They are removed using polyp forceps under general anaesthesia but they may recur.

UTERINE FIBROIDS

Fibroids or leiomyomata are the commonest tumours of the female genital tract and are present in at least 20% of women over the age of 30 years. Their aetiology is unknown but their growth is oestrogen-dependent and they regress after the menopause. Fibroids are associated with nulliparity in Caucasian women and they are more prevalent in Negro women.

Fibroids are mainly derived from smooth muscle but also contain some fibrous tissue elements. They form well-defined tumours with a false capsule and may be found in various sites: intramural fibroids lie within the uterine wall, subserous fibroids project from the peritoneal surface of the uterus, and submucous fibroids encroach on the uterine cavity, sometimes distorting it and increasing its surface area. Subserous fibroids may become pedunculated and a submucous fibroid may become extruded to form a fibroid polyp. Only 2% of fibroids arise in the cervix.

Fibroids are usually multiple and vary in size from seedlings to large tumours. They may undergo various types of degenerative changes:

Hyaline degeneration. This is the commonest change and it occurs as the fibroid outgrows its blood supply. Areas liquefy and cysts form.

Calcification. This occurs in postmenopausal women.

Infection. Subserous or pedunculated fibroids may become infected by spread from adjacent structures. Ascending infection may complicate submucous fibroids.

Red degeneration. This occurs during pregnancy when the blood supply is insufficient to support growth of the fibroid; the cut section of the fibroid appears red.

Malignant change is rare ($< 0.5\%$ of fibroids) and may be suspected when there is rapid or painful enlargement of fibroids.

Assessment

The majority of fibroids are asymptomatic and are detected at routine pelvic examination. The commonest symptom is menorrhagia which is particularly associated with submucous fibroids. Some women present with abdominal distension and others complain of pressure symptoms such as increased frequency of micturition and stress incontinence. Pain is an unusual feature but occasionally fibroids present as an acute abdomen following torsion of a pedunculated fibroid or haemorrhage into a large fibroid. Fibroids do not cause infertility unless they are obstructing the cornua of the uterus.

Pelvic examination reveals an enlarged and often irregular uterus which may be palpable per abdomen. The main differential diagnosis is from ovarian tumours where the uterus should be detected separately from the pelvic mass. The presence of ascites is highly suggestive of ovarian pathology. In practice, it may be difficult to distinguish between the two clinically.

Investigations

Ultrasonography may be useful to distinguish between uterine and ovarian pathology. Abnormal vaginal bleeding should not be assumed to be due to fibroids and other pathology should be excluded. A cervical smear should be performed and the patient should have an endometrial biopsy.

Blood tests may reveal iron deficiency anaemia but large fibroids are rarely associated with polycythaemia (due to erythropoietin production).

Treatment

Conservative management

Conservative management is appropriate in the following situations:

1. Uterus smaller than 16 weeks' gestation
2. Asymptomatic
3. During pregnancy
4. Menopause approaching
5. Fertility required.

Medical treatment of fibroids using GnRH analogues has produced disappointing results. Fibroids regress during treatment but rapidly regrow when therapy is discontinued. Duration of treatment is limited by bone loss due to oestrogen deficiency.

Surgery

Surgery is indicated in the following situations:

1. Fibroids causing symptoms
2. Uterus > 16 weeks' size
3. Rapid growth in fibroids
4. Recurrent abortion/fibroid-related complications in previous pregnancy (see below)
5. Diagnosis uncertain.

Hysterectomy is the definitive procedure. Myomectomy can be technically difficult and regrowth of fibroids after this procedure is common. Myomectomy should be reserved for women who wish to retain fertility and for those who decline hysterectomy. Myomectomy does not usually prejudice outcome of future pregnancies and scar rupture is rare.

Fibroids in pregnancy

Fibroids may be detected for the first time in pregnancy. They may cause the uterus to feel large for dates. They do not usually influence the outcome of the pregnancy but they may be associated with some complications:

1. Recurrent abortion: submucous fibroids distort the uterine cavity and may be associated with repeated early pregnancy loss
2. Pain: red degeneration may occur in large fibroids causing pain and localized uterine tenderness; treatment is by rest and analgesia; torsion of a pedunculated fibroid may occur
3. Malpresentations/abnormal lie
4. Obstructed labour (rare)
5. Postpartum haemorrhage.

Surgical treatment of fibroids is not undertaken during pregnancy except in the rare situation when a pedunculated fibroid undergoes torsion.

THE OVARIES

Functional cysts of the ovaries are common and they usually cause no symptoms. Follicular cysts are rarely > 5 cm in diameter and are usually diagnosed by ultrasound in women with anovulatory cycles and those receiving fertility treatment. Corpus lutein cysts are associated with short periods of secondary amenorrhoea followed by heavier than usual bleeding. Multiple theca lutein cysts are characteristically associated with trophoblastic disease and hyperstimulation associated with fertility treatment. Functional cysts usually resolve spontaneously and should be followed up by ultrasonography. Persistent cysts can be aspirated via the laparoscope. Cytological examination of the cyst fluid should always be performed.

ENDOMETRIOSIS

See Pelvic pain.

OVARIAN NEOPLASMS

See Gynaecological neoplasia.

15. Gynaecological neoplasia

A. Rodin

Neoplasia of the female genital tract is common and may be benign or malignant. At present in England and Wales, one woman in 20 will develop a gynaecological malignancy and one woman in 40 will die of the disease. Cancer of the ovary is the most common gynaecological cancer.

Expectations of the examiners

Candidates are expected to understand the natural history of the common gynaecological neoplasms and to know the principles of their management. An appreciation of the role of screening is of particular importance to the general practitioner.

THE VULVA

Carcinoma of the vulva may be preceded by skin changes. There are three categories:

1. Vulval dystrophies
2. Vulval intraepithelial neoplasia (VIN)
3. Human papilloma virus infection.

The chronic vulval dystrophies may be premalignant in the presence of nuclear atypia (increased mitotic activity, irregularity of nuclear size and shape and nuclear hyperchromasia, see Benign conditions of the female genital tracts Ch. 14). In these circumstances the histological appearance may satisfy the criteria for VIN (see below) and there is some overlap between VIN and the chronic vulval dystrophies. Human papilloma virus infection is common and has been implicated as a possible cause of VIN.

VULVAL INTRAEPITHELIAL NEOPLASIA

In the past, the premalignant changes of the vulva were known as carcinoma in situ or Bowen's disease. The nomenclature has now changed and they are classified as VIN 1, 2 and 3.

VIN 1. The epidermis is thickened and nuclear atypia is confined to the basal third of the epithelium.

VIN 2. Marked nuclear atypia in the lower half of the epithelium.

VIN 3. Carcinoma in situ. Marked nuclear atypia extending through the full thickness of the epithelium.

VIN cannot be detected by cytology. Colposcopy has been used but diagnosis depends on histological examination of skin biopsies. VIN may be associated with other genital tract neoplasia (e.g. cervical intraepithelial neoplasia).

Treatment

1. Local destruction
    a. Laser vaporization
    b. Cryosurgery
    c. 5-Fluorouracil cream.
2. Surgical excision
    a. Wide excision
    b. Simple vulvectomy
    c. Skinning vulvectomy.

Treatment depends on the site and size of the area of neoplasia, the histology and the preferences of the gynaecologist. Recurrences do occur and follow-up is essential.

CARCINOMA OF THE VULVA

Carcinoma of the vulva is rare and accounts for 3–5% of all genital tract malignancies. This cancer mainly affects women in their late 70s and is of unknown aetiology.

Pathology

Most carcinomas of the vulva are squamous (85%) and the remainder are melanomas, carcinomas of the Bartholin's gland and other rare tumours. The majority occur on the labia and spread occurs via the lymphatics initially to the inguinal and femoral nodes, and then to the deep pelvic nodes.

Assessment

Over two-thirds of patients present with a history of chronic pruritus vulvae and they may also have noticed a lump or ulcer. The general medical condition of the woman must be carefully assessed as the majority of patients are elderly.

Staging

Stage I.   Lesion confined to vulva and maximum diameter 2 cm. No suspicious groin nodes.

Stage II.   Lesion confined to vulva with diameter > 2 cm. No suspicious groin nodes.

Stage III.   Lesion extends beyond vulva with no suspicious nodes,
  or
  Lesion of any size confined to vulva with suspicious nodes.

Stage IV.   Lesion of any size with obviously positive nodes,
  or
  Lesion involving rectum, bladder, urethra or bone,
  or
  All cases with pelvic or distant spread.

This staging system has limitations and it fails to take into account the site or histology of the tumour. The majority of patients present with stage I disease.

Management

Radical vulvectomy and bilateral groin node dissection is the treatment of choice in the majority of cases. For very early stage I lesions, some advocate wide local excision. In advanced cases, more radical surgery may be indicated and this may involve pelvic exenteration.

Survival

This is closely related to tumour stage and presence of lymph node involvement. The five-year survival for node negative stage I cases is about 95%.

THE VAGINA

Vaginal carcinoma is rarer than carcinoma of the vulva and detailed discussion of this tumour is beyond the scope of this book. Ninety per cent of tumours are squamous cell carcinomas and most patients present in the sixth and seventh decades with abnormal vaginal bleeding and discharge. Clear cell adenocarcinomas are associated with in utero exposure to diethylstilboestrol.

VAGINAL INTRAEPITHELIAL NEOPLASIA (VAIN)

This condition is diagnosed by cytology or colposcopy. It usually occurs in conjunction with and often in continuity with cervical intraepithelial neoplasia. The histological features of VAIN are identical to those of cervical intraepithelial neoplasia. Treatment is by local ablation (laser vaporization, cryocautery, electrodiathermy and surgical excision is rarely required.

THE CERVIX

Squamous cell carcinoma of the cervix is preventable if the premalignant stages are detected and treated, however, the incidence of these pre-malignant changes and invasive carcinoma is increasing. Carcinoma of the cervix is more common in parous women and risk may be increased in long-term pill users and in smokers. The most important factor is sexual behaviour and an early age of first coitus increases a woman's risk of developing this condition. Nuns have a low incidence while prostitutes have a high incidence. Carcinoma of the cervix is a venereal disease and a number of factors transmitted during coitus have been proposed as possible causative agents, including smegma and herpes simplex virus. Human papilloma virus (HPV) is currently under suspicion and types 16 and 18 have been found in cervical cancer tissue and in association with cervical intraepithelial neoplasia, but a causative relationship is yet to be established.

CERVICAL INTRAEPITHELIAL NEOPLASIA (CIN)

CIN is an epithelial abnormality of the cervix or dysplasia which is classified into three grades; CIN 1 corresponds to mild dysplasia, CIN 2 to moderate dysplasia and CIN 3 includes severe dysplasia and carcinoma in

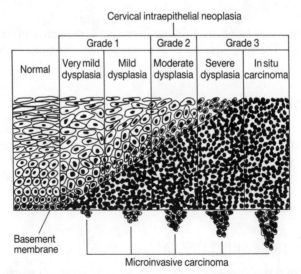

Fig. 15.1 Precursors to invasive carcinoma of the cervix. The diagram illustrates abnormal changes in the cervical epithelium in CIN 1–3. Microinvasion is shown as crossing the basement membrane.

situ. Dysplasia is a histological term and describes a lesion in which part of the thickness of the epithelium is replaced by cells showing varying degrees of nuclear atypia. Dyskaryosis is a cytological diagnosis. Figure 15.1 shows the precursors to invasive carcinoma of the cervix.

CIN 1.   Nuclear atypia confined to the basal third of the epithelium.
CIN 2.   Nuclear atypia in the basal two-thirds of the epithelium with abnormalities more marked than in CIN 1.
CIN 3.   Nuclear abnormalities throughout the whole thickness of the epithelium.

CIN 1 may regress to normality but any degree of CIN may progress to carcinoma of the cervix.

Screening for CIN is by cervical cytology (see Screening for gynaecological neoplasia p. 122). Colposcopically directed biopsy provides a histological diagnosis.

Treatment

1. Local ablative techniques
   a. Cryosurgery
   b. 'Cold' coagulation
   c. Laser
   d. Diathermy
2. Large loop excision of transformation zone
3. Cone biopsy
   a. Surgical
   b. Laser
   c. Loop
4. Hysterectomy.

The following criteria must be fulfilled before a local ablative method is used: 1. the whole lesion must be visible; 2. there must be no suspicion of invasion; 3. follow-up must be adequate and involve colposcopy and cervical cytology which is performed annually.

CARCINOMA OF THE CERVIX

The incidence and mortality from carcinoma of the cervix is increasing. Approximately 4000 new cases of invasive carcinoma of the cervix occur in England and Wales annually. Half of these cases present at an early stage but 50% of women with invasive disease will die within five years of diagnosis. The peak incidence of carcinoma of the cervix is in the 50s.

Pathology

In most cases, cervical carcinoma passes through a premalignant phase before becoming invasive. This precancerous stage is of variable duration. Squamous cell tumours comprise 90% of tumours and originate within the transformation zone. The remainder are adenocarcinomas. Spread occurs by either direct extension into adjacent structures or by lymphatic permeation. Renal failure following bilateral ureteric obstruction is a common cause of death.

Assessment

Patients may present with postcoital bleeding, intermenstrual bleeding or an offensive vaginal discharge. A certain number will be detected by routine screening. The diagnosis is confirmed by histological examination of a cervical biopsy.

Further investigations are performed to check for spread of disease and include a chest X-ray and intravenous urogram. Lymphangiography or CT scanning may be useful to detect lymphatic involvement, however these techniques have their limitations.

Staging

Carcinoma of the cervix is staged clinically. Traditionally the patient is examined under anaesthesia when cervical biopsy, endometrial currettage and cystoscopy are performed.

> *Stage I.*   Carcinoma confined to the cervix.
> Ia. Microinvasive carcinoma.
> Ib. All other cases.
> *Stage II.*   Carcinoma extends beyond the cervix but not to the pelvic side wall. Carcinoma may involve the upper two-thirds of the vagina.
> IIa. No obvious parametrial involvement.
> IIb. Obvious parametrial involvement.
> *Stage III.*   Carcinoma extends to the pelvic side wall. The lower one-third of the vagina may be involved. Hydronephrosis or non-functioning kidney.
> *Stage IV.*   Carcinoma extending beyond the true pelvis or involving the mucosa of the bladder or rectum.

The definition of microinvasion is controversial and depends on careful histological examination of biopsy material.

Management

Microinvasive disease can be treated without radical surgery or radiotherapy. Hysterectomy is generally advised but in some cases cone biopsy may be considered adequate treatment, particularly in a young woman who wants a pregnancy.

With early stage disease (Ib or IIa) there is a choice between radical surgery or radiotherapy. Similar survival rates are achieved by these methods, however there is less morbidity associated with surgical treatment and this is favoured in the 'young and fit' woman. Radiotherapy is associated with urological and gastrointestinal complications and ovarian irradiation results in a premature menopause. Radiation vaginitis results in stenosis and sexual dysfunction is common. The object of Wertheim's radical hysterectomy is to remove the uterus, Fallopian tubes, parametrium, upper third of vagina and the pelvic lymph nodes. The ovaries are sometimes conserved. The main hazards of radical surgery are the risks of the operation itself, pulmonary embolism and ureteric fistula formation.

There is no consensus about the most appropriate management of advanced or recurrent cervical cancer. Radiotherapy is commonly used and pelvic exenteration may be performed in selected cases. The role of chemotherapy is being evaluated.

Survival

Results obtained by surgery and radiotherapy in early stage disease are very similar and five-year survival figures are about 80%. The finding of involved lymph nodes at surgery is associated with a poor prognosis.

THE BODY OF THE UTERUS

CARCINOMA OF THE ENDOMETRIUM

Endometrial carcinoma is primarily a disease of postmenopausal women. Peak incidence is between 55 and 70 years and only 5% of cases occur in women < 40 years. The incidence of this neoplasm is increasing for reasons that are poorly understood. Obesity, nulliparity and a late menopause are all associated with carcinoma of the endometrium and patients are more likely to be diabetic or hypertensive. Unopposed oestrogen replacement therapy in women with a uterus increases the risk of endometrial carcinoma.

Pathology

Endometrial carcinoma may be preceded by endometrial hyperplasia or by an endometrial polyp. Most tumours are adenocarcinomas which tend to be slow growing. They spread by direct extension and then via the lymphatics and the bloodstream.

Assessment

Over 90% of women with carcinoma of the endometrium present with postmenopausal vaginal bleeding. Some have a blood-stained purulent discharge due to a pyometra and a small number are asymptomatic. Although only 10% of women who present with postmenopausal bleeding have carcinoma of the endometrium, it is essential that this diagnosis is excluded in all cases and endometrial curettage is mandatory.

On vaginal examination, the uterus may be enlarged. Diagnosis is by histological examination of endometrial curettings. Hysteroscopy is being increasingly used in the assessment of women with postmenopausal bleeding.

Staging

Stage I. Carcinoma confined to the body of the uterus.
    Ia. Uterine cavity 8 cm or less.
    Ib. Uterine cavity > 8 cm.
Stage II. Carcinoma involving the body of the uterus and the cervix but not extending beyond the uterus.
Stage III. Carcinoma extending beyond the uterus but not beyond the true pelvis.
Stage IV. Carcinoma extending outside the true pelvis or involving the mucosa of the bladder or rectum.

Management

The mainstay of treatment is total abdominal hysterectomy and bilateral salpingo-oophorectomy. Adjuvant therapy may be given depending on the depth of myometrial invasion and tumour differentiation.

Radiotherapy is commonly used and progestogen therapy is recommended for advanced or recurrent disease. It may also be beneficial in early stage disease.

Survival

Factors influencing survival in endometrial carcinoma are age at diagnosis, stage of disease, pathological type and degree of differentiation of the lesion and the depth of myometrial invasion. Five-year survival for stage I disease is 75% and it is < 10% for stage IV disease.

THE OVARIES

CARCINOMA OF THE OVARY

Cancer of the ovary is most prevalent in industrialized societies and tends to affect the upper social classes. Peak incidence is between the ages of 60–70 years and it carries the worst prognosis of all the malignancies of the female genital tract. Cancer of the ovary has an incidence of 14 per 100 000 women in the UK. Women with a history of carcinoma of the ovary amongst first degree relatives have an increased risk of developing the disease themselves. Pregnancy and oral contraceptives reduce the risks of carcinoma of the ovary.

Pathology

Neoplastic disease of the ovary includes a variety of histological types which can be classified as follows:

1. Epithelial tumours
2. Germ cell tumours
3. Sex cord tumours
4. Nonspecific mesenchymal tumours
5. Secondary tumours.

Ninety per cent of ovarian tumours are epithelial in origin, derived from the serosal covering of the ovary. Within this group there are a number of histological types: serous, mucinous, endometrioid, Brenner and clear cell. Each of these neoplasms can exist in a benign or malignant form and the malignant forms are collectively known as adenocarcinoma of the ovary.

The commonest germ cell tumour is the benign cystic teratoma or dermoid cyst. This is derived from totipotent germ cells and may contain a variety of tissues including teeth, bone, cartilage, muscle, thyroid tissue and nervous tissue. The cavity of the cyst often contains sebum and hair. Dermoid cysts are usually benign and are most common during re-productive life. In about 20% of cases they are bilateral.

Sex cord tumours are rare and include granulosa and theca cell tumours. These tumours usually secrete oestrogens and the effects of this depend on the age of the patient.

Spread of carcinoma of the ovary to the contralateral ovary and uterus is common. Transperitoneal seeding occurs to the pelvic peritoneum, omentum and other abdominal viscera. There may be lymphatic spread to the pelvic nodes and para-aortic nodes with distant spread to the media-stinal and supraclavicular nodes.

Assessment

Many ovarian tumours cause no symptoms and as a result, 75% of cases of carcinoma of the ovary present at an advanced stage (stage III or IV—see below). Even when symptoms are present they may be nonspecific. Pain is uncommon but may follow torsion, rupture or haemorrhage into an ovarian neoplasm. Increasing abdominal girth may be due to tumour bulk or the presence of ascites. Compression of adjacent structures may cause symptoms such as increased frequency of micturition. Meig's syndrome is a rare condition in which there is ascites and a pleural effusion associated with a benign ovarian fibroma.

Ultrasonography is useful in the preoperative investigation of a pelvic mass but staging is based on findings at clinical examination and laparotomy.

Staging

Stage I. Tumour confined to the ovaries.
Ia. Confined to one ovary; no ascites.
Ib. Confined to both ovaries; no ascites.
Ic. Tumour confined to the ovaries with ascites or positive peritoneal washings.
Stage II. Tumour involving one or both ovaries with pelvic extension.
IIa. Spread to the uterus and/or tubes.
IIb. Spread to other pelvic tissues.
IIc. Stage IIa or IIb with ascites or positive peritoneal washings.
Stage III. Tumour involving one or both ovaries with intraperitoneal spread outside the pelvis or tumour limited to the pelvis with extension to the small bowel or omentum.
Stage IV. Tumour involving one or both ovaries with distant spread.

Management

The aim of primary surgery is to stage the tumour and to reduce the tumour bulk as much as possible. Total abdominal hysterectomy, bilateral oophorectomy and omentectomy are performed. Chemotherapy has improved survival particularly in more advanced disease. The role of second look laparotomy or laparoscopy in the management of women with carcinoma of the ovary is controversial.

Survival

Five-year survival for early stage disease is about 65%. Prognosis for women with more advanced disease is worse and only 5–12% of women with stage III disease survive to five years. Overall five-year survival is 30%.

SCREENING FOR GYNAECOLOGICAL NEOPLASIA

The prognosis for women with all gynaecological malignancies is improved if detection and treatment occurs at an early stage. Better still, malignancy can be prevented if the disease is found in its precancerous stage and adequately treated.

Screening tests should be simple to apply to an at risk group and they must have a high sensitivity with few false negative or false positive results. Ultimately, the cost effectiveness of a screening programme must be demonstrated.

SCREENING FOR CARCINOMA OF THE CERVIX

Cancer of the cervix is preceded by a premalignant stage (CIN) which is of variable duration. Screening is aimed at detecting and treating women with CIN before malignancy develops and programmes may be systematic or opportunistic. The systematic approach involves regular screening and rescreening of all women considered at risk. Opportunistic programmes rely on screening women when they attend for other forms of medical care, e.g. at family planning clinics and at postnatal checks.

The accessibility of the cervix allows samples of cells to be taken periodically and cytological examination is performed. This test was developed by Papanicolaou in 1943. The technique for taking a cervical smear is simple and various types of spatula are available. Brushes allow sampling from the endocervical canal.

In 1966, in the UK a programme was adopted that involved five-yearly screening of women over 35 years of age. Women under this age were not encouraged to attend for screening. The rising incidence of cervical cancer in young women and the realization that the majority of women with invasive cancer had never had a smear led to a review of the screening programme.

The Department of Health currently recommends that all women who have been sexually active should be screened at five-yearly intervals. In addition, women should be screened when first presenting for contraceptive advice.

The choice of a five-year interval is based on the belief that there is a latent period of at least 10 years between the development of a positive smear and presentation with invasive cancer. However, the degree of 'protection' against cervical cancer given by a negative smear falls steadily after only three years and the screening interval should be reduced to three years.

In areas where there are comprehensive and systematic screening programmes, there has been a reduction in incidence of invasive carcinoma and a fall in mortality.

CARCINOMA OF THE OVARY

Early detection of this malignancy is difficult because it is often asymptomatic, it is not preceded by a premalignant stage and there is no readily identifiable high-risk group. Screening by vaginal examination, pelvic ultrasonography and the use of tumour markers (e.g. CA125) is currently being evaluated. The role of prophylactic oophorectomy in the prevention of carcinoma of the ovary is controversial.

16. The menopause, hormone replacement therapy and premenstrual syndrome

A. Rodin

Expectations of the examiners

The candidate is expected to understand the basic physiology of the menopause. A knowledge of the long-term effects of the menopause is required and a detailed understanding of the management of women on hormone replacement therapy is needed. The candidate should have a basic understanding of the premenstrual syndrome and the management of women with this condition.

THE MENOPAUSE

Definition

The menopause is defined as the cessation of menstruation and it marks the end of a woman's reproductive potential.

Interesting facts

The average age of the menopause in the UK is 51 years. Interest in menopause-related problems has grown due to the increase in mean female life expectancy, which is now 82 years (in the UK).

The average woman spends 38% of her life after the menopause and in the UK postmenopausal women number more than nine million and comprise 18% of the total population. The short and long-term problems associated with the menopause cause significant morbidity and mortality and have important economic implications. Women who do not suffer the 'acute' symptoms of the menopause remain at risk of long-term complications.

Physiology

The menopause is the result of ovarian failure and it is preceded by a transition phase known as the climacteric which is of variable duration. The climacteric is characterized by increasing resistance of the ovarian follicles to stimulation by the gonadotrophins. Total oestrogen output by the ovaries declines and therefore gonadotrophin levels increase. Anovulation becomes more frequent and as a result progesterone deficiency occurs; this may lead to prolonged or irregular vaginal bleeding. These changes commence 10 to 15 years before the menopause and some women complain of symptoms of oestrogen deficiency during the climacteric.

Prior to the menopause, the main oestrogen is 17 beta-oestradiol which is secreted by the ovaries. This is converted to oestrone which has one-tenth the potency of 17 beta-oestradiol, and then to oestriol. In the post-menopausal woman, ovarian 17 beta-oestradiol production ceases and oestrone becomes the primary oestrogen. The major source of oestrone after the menopause is the peripheral conversion in adipose tissue of androstenedione which is produced by the adrenal cortex (70%) and the ovary (30%). After the menopause, the ovary continues to secrete androgens, mainly testosterone and androstenedione. FSH and LH levels plateau 2 to 3 years after the menopause and begin to decline after 5 to 10 years.

The effects of oestrogen deficiency

Oestrogen deficiency is responsible for the characteristic features of the menopausal syndrome. Most systems are affected but the manifestations vary between individuals. Vasomotor instability affects 75% of women and 25% are severely affected. Hot flushes and night sweats may continue for more than five years in 25% of women. Flushes can be socially disabling and may interfere with daily activities while night sweats result in interrupted sleep and progressive fatigue. The mechanism of menopausal vasomotor instability is uncertain but a hypothalamic mechanism has been suggested.

Atrophy occurs in all oestrogen sensitive tissues, notably the urogenital tract, breasts and skin. In the vagina, there is flattening and thinning of the epithelium which may result in atrophic vaginitis. Loss of glycogen from the epithelial cells leads to the disappearance of the lactic acid forming Döderlein's bacilli and as a consequence, the vagina becomes alkaline. The bladder and urethra, which are lined by transitional epithelium, undergo similar changes to the vagina. The supporting structures of the genital tract lose tone and prolapse may become apparent. Breasts become atrophic with a reduction in adipose tissue and lobules.

The psychological effects of the menopause may be the direct result of oestrogen deficiency on the central nervous system or they may be precipitated by distressing physical symptoms or life events.

The long-term consequences of the menopause are:

Osteoporosis. Postmenopausal osteoporosis is a major health care problem. The important fracture sites are the vertebrae and the femoral neck. Twenty-five per cent of women over 60 will suffer vertebral crush

Table 16.1 Common presenting symptoms of the menopause.

Physical	Psychological
Hot flushes	Depression
Night sweats	Anxiety/panic attacks
Exhaustion	Irritability
Joint pains	Lethargy
Dysuria	Poor memory
Vaginal dryness	Poor concentration
Dyspareunia	Decreased libido

fractures. The incidence of fractured neck of femur is increasing although the reasons for this trend are unclear. Twenty per cent of women who suffer this type of fracture die from complications and many of those that survive never return to full mobility.

Following the menopause, bone mineral is lost from the skeleton at an accelerated rate for about five years and then becomes more gradual. Women who have an early menopause are at greater risk of osteoporosis in later life.

Other risk factors include smoking, alcohol abuse and steroid treatment. Thin Caucasians are at higher risk and family history is also thought to be important.

Cardiovascular disease. Premenopausal women have a lower risk of cardiovascular disease compared to men of the same age group. This is thought to be due to the effect of oestrogen on the lipid profile (raises HDL-cholesterol and lowers LDL-cholesterol). Oestrogen is also an arterial vasodilator. Following the menopause the protective effect of oestrogen is lost and the prevalence of cardiovascular disease in women increases.

Assessment

The diagnosis is usually straightforward and is based on the history. Common presenting symptoms are listed in Table 16.1.

It is important to elicit how the symptoms are interfering with everyday activities and relationships. Diagnosis may be less obvious in women who have premature ovarian failure and in women who have undergone hysterectomy with conservation of the ovaries. A medical history should exclude contraindications to hormone replacement therapy. Smoking should be discouraged. General physical examination should include breast examination and height, weight and blood pressure should be recorded. Pelvic examination should include a cervical smear if indicated.

Investigations

Blood tests are rarely helpful but in cases where the diagnosis is in doubt, measure serum gonadotrophins and/or oestradiol. Oestradiol < 70 pmol/l and FSH/LH > 15 i.u./l are found in menopausal women. Endometrial biopsy is not performed as a routine but it is mandatory in women with postmenopausal bleeding or irregular bleeding. Mammography should be offered to women over 50 years.

Noninvasive methods are now available for the measurement of bone density in the spine and femoral neck. Dual photon absorptiometry and CT scanning are both in use.

Treatment

Nonhormonal preparations have been used to treat menopausal symptoms but they are generally ineffective and provide no protection from the long-term effects of the menopause. Hormone replacement therapy (HRT) is the most appropriate treatment for women with menopause-related problems. The decision to commence HRT should be made after full discussion with the patient.

Indications for HRT include:

1. Menopause-related symptoms
2. Early menopause
3. Prevention of osteoporosis
4. Cardiovascular protection.

Contraindications to oestrogen replacement therapy:

1. Carcinoma of the breast
2. Carcinoma of the endometrium
3. Malignant melanoma (if appeared during pregnancy/on pill)
4. Liver disease (porphyria, active hepatitis).

Hypertension is not a contraindication to therapy but blood pressure should be stabilized before HRT is commenced. Women with a history of thromboembolic disease can be given HRT but it is often advisable to refer women with a complicated medical history to the local menopause clinic.

Oestrogen therapy

'Natural' oestrogens (17 beta-oestradiol, oestradiol valerate, conjugated equine oestrogens) are favoured for HRT rather than synthetic oestrogens which are found in the combined oral contraceptive preparations. Oestrogen should be given continuously and may be administered orally or parenterally. The pharmacodynamics and biochemical effects of exogenous oestrogens can vary markedly with the route of administration. Oral therapy is the most widely used. Oestrogen delivered by this route first passes through the liver. This has several effects:

1. Hepatic metabolism removes a large proportion of a given dose.

2. Oestrogen may influence the synthesis of various hepatic products and this may have beneficial or adverse effects; oral oestrogen favourably alters the HDL/LDL ratio by elevating plasma HDL-cholesterol; oral therapy may increase renin substrate production and a parenteral route of administration may be more appropriate in hypertensives; similarly antithrombin III production may be depressed, and parenteral administration may be advisable in women with clotting disorders.
3. Concurrent drug therapy (e.g. with anticonvulsants) may result in induction of hepatic enzymes leading to rapid inactivation of oestrogen.

The parenteral route avoids the first pass effect and is particularly suitable for hypertensives and women with a history of thromboembolic disease. It is a convenient method following hysterectomy. Subcutaneous implants of oestradiol (50 mg) are inserted under local anaesthesia into the anterior abdominal wall or buttock. Testosterone (100 mg) may be added to improve libido; testosterone cannot be taken orally. The procedure is repeated every six months. Vaginal administration of oestrogen creams results in blood levels comparable to those seen after oral therapy and endometrial hyperplasia may occur with long-term use. Oestrogen can now be administered transdermally via skin patches which are convenient and effective.

Progestogen therapy

Prolonged administration of oestrogens to postmenopausal women is associated with an increase in incidence of endometrial carcinoma. This risk can be avoided by adding a progestogen for 12 days each calendar month. Side-effects can be reduced by using the minimum dose of progestogen.

Unwanted effects of progestogen are: 1. withdrawal bleeding; 2. 'premenstrual' symptoms; 3. alterations in the lipid profile which may counteract the favourable effect of oestrogen.

Approaches to treatment

For the purposes of treatment, women can be classified into two groups: those who have a uterus; and those who have previously undergone hysterectomy. Women should be fully counselled before starting treatment and they should be warned about common side-effects.

Oral therapy is appropriate for women with a uterus. Continuous oestrogen should be given with the addition of a progestogen for 12 days each month. The majority of women will have withdrawal bleeds on this regime and some will experience breast tenderness.

In women with hypertension or a history of thromboembolic disease, it may be preferable to administer oestrogen parenterally and to give a progestogen for 12 days each month (progestogens cannot be administered parenterally).

Women who have had a hysterectomy do not need progestagens.

Follow-up of women on HRT

Women should be reviewed three months after treatment is commenced. Symptoms should be discussed and enquiries should be made about patterns of vaginal bleeding. Weight and blood pressure should be recorded at each visit. Subsequently, women should be reviewed every six months. Smears should be taken as necessary and annual breast examination should be performed. Mammography can be repeated every 2–3 years. Unscheduled vaginal bleeding must be investigated promptly with an endometrial biopsy.

There is no consensus about the optimum duration of hormone replacement therapy. To obtain significant protection from osteoporotic fractures, a minimum course of five years' treatment is recommended.

Advantages of hormone replacement therapy

1. Relief from menopausal symptoms.
2. Prevention of bone demineralization; oestrogen therapy halts bone loss and protects against osteoporotic fractures. It is most effective if it is commenced shortly after the menopause to avoid the period of accelerated bone loss. The minimum bone-sparing dosages of oestradiol valerate and conjugated oestrogens are 2 mg and 0.625 mg respectively.
3. Evidence is accumulating that oestrogen therapy protects against cardiovascular disease.

HRT and cancer

Concerns about the link between HRT and cancer seem to be largely unfounded. Recent evidence suggests that the addition of cyclical progestogens to oestrogen replacement therapy reduces the risk of endometrial cancer to below that in an untreated population. There is no association between HRT and carcinoma of the cervix and ovary. Epidemiological evidence about the effect of HRT on the incidence of carcinoma of the breast is unclear but some studies suggest a small increase in risk with prolonged use.

SUMMARY

The average woman spends more than one-third of her life after the menopause. The long-term sequelae of the menopause have important medical implications. The benefits of HRT in improving menopausal symptoms, preventing osteoporosis and reducing the incidence of cardiovascular disease are well recognized.

PREMENSTRUAL SYNDROME

Definition

Distressing physical and psychological symptoms which occur during the premenstrual phase of the menstrual/ovarian cycle and regress at the onset of menstruation.

Interesting facts

The premenstrual syndrome (PMS) was first described by Frank in 1931. He reported a small group of women with tension, depression and irritability occurring 7–10 days before menstruation and relieved by the onset of 'the menstrual flow'. This condition remains poorly understood. Estimates of the prevalence of PMS in the general population vary from 5% to 95%.

Pathophysiology

The aetiology of PMS is unknown. It is likely that PMS is not a homogeneous condition but it is due to a combination of physical, psychological, genetic and environmental factors. A variety of mechanisms have been proposed in PMS but they remain unproven. Popular hypotheses include progesterone deficiency, fluid retention, vitamin deficiency, hypoglycaemia or defective prostaglandin metabolism. The link between PMS and cyclical ovarian activity is certain and the condition characteristically commences after pregnancy or discontinuation of the combined contraceptive pill with the resumption of ovarian activity.

Assessment

Diagnosis is based on the history. Symptoms are many and varied and any body system may be involved. Patterns of symptoms vary between women and the severity of symptoms may vary from cycle to cycle. Common symptoms are listed in Table 16.2.

In addition, there may be behavioural changes and pre-existing medical

Table 16.2 Symptoms of premenstrual syndrome.

Physical	Psychological
Breast discomfort	Irritability
Bloating	Anxiety
Weight gain	Tension
Acne	Depression
Headache	Insomnia
Pelvic pain	Change in libido
Change in bowel habit	Poor concentration

Table 16.3   Treatments used in premenstrual syndrome.

Drug treatment
  Hormonal
    Progesterone
    Combined pill
    LHRH analogues
    Oestradiol implants
    Danazol
  Non-hormonal
    Diuretics
    Vitamins B6, A, E,
    Bromocryptine
    Prostaglandin synthetase
    Inhibitors
    Psychoactive drugs
    Gamma-linolenic acid

Psychological
  Psychotherapy
  Hypnosis

Other
  Diet
  Acupuncture
  Bilateral oophorectomy
  Radiation menopause

conditions such as epilepsy, asthma or herpes may be exacerbated. If the history is suggestive of PMS, confirmatory evidence can be obtained by prospectively assessing symptoms over three cycles. Various methods have been used ranging from self-grading of severity of symptoms to the use of visual analogue scales.

Blood tests are of no value in the diagnosis of PMS.

Treatment

A variety of approaches have been used and these are summarized in Table 16.3.

The placebo response in PMS may exceed 90% and consequently it is difficult to prove the effectiveness of any active treatment. The choice of first-line treatment will be influenced by the severity of symptoms. In mild cases, vitamin B6 or gamma-linolenic acid may be helpful. The combined contraceptive pill or dydrogesterone 10 mg b.d. on days 12 to 26 of the cycle can be prescribed for moderately affected women.

In severe cases, inhibition of the ovarian cycle is the approach of choice. This can be achieved by using subcutaneous oestradiol implants combined with cyclical oral progestogen to prevent the development of endometrial hyperplasia. LHRH analogues are extremely effective but because of the suppression of ovarian oestrogen production they are not appropriate for long-term use.

If single symptoms predominate, it may be preferable to try a therapy aimed at alleviating that specific complaint; for example, bromocriptine for breast pain and diuretics for bloating. Counselling or psychotherapy may be beneficial in women with PMS.

SUMMARY

PMS is associated with cyclical ovarian activity and does not occur before puberty, during pregnancy or after the menopause. Most women experience adverse symptoms prior to menstruation. The aetiology of PMS is unknown and treatments are non-specific. In severe cases, ovarian suppression is the treatment of choice.

17. Urinary incontinence

J. Rymer

Expectations of the examiners

The candidate will be expected to have a basic knowledge of the physiology of micturition, and the various types of incontinence. In particular, the candidate should be able to distinguish between stress and urge incontinence, and manage appropriately. In the clinical examination the candidate could be asked to demonstrate stress incontinence as described below.

STRESS INCONTINENCE

Definition

Involuntary loss of urine coinciding with a rise in intra-abdominal pressure (e.g. laughing, coughing, jumping).

Pathophysiology

Control of micturition depends on two main factors:

1. A competent sphincter mechanism able to resist the changes in intra-abdominal pressure
2. The capacity to inhibit a bladder contraction until it is convenient to micturate.

Urine leakage occurs when the intravesical pressure exceeds the maximum urethral pressure. Most commonly the urethral 'occlusive forces' have been diminished by childbirth trauma and/or menopausal atrophy, and this deficiency is aggravated by descent of the proximal third of the urethra below the level of the pelvic floor (Fig. 17.1).

Assessment

History

History is important to determine whether this is pure stress incontinence or whether an element of urgency is present. Chronic constipation, chronic

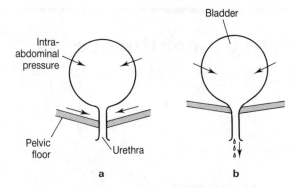

Fig. 17.1   Stress incontinence. **a**. Normally an increase in intra-abdominal pressure will be transmitted to the bladder and to the urethra, thus maintaining continence. **b**. If there is an alteration in the position of the bladder neck and most of the urethra is below the pelvic floor then an increase in intra-abdominal pressure will increase the intravesical pressure but not the urethral pressure, so that urine will be lost.

bronchitis, smoking and diuretics are associated with stress incontinence and should be specifically asked about. Classically the incontinence occurs synchronously with the rise in intra-abdominal pressure. Most patients find incontinence a social and hygienic problem.

Examination

General and abdominal examination should be performed. To assess the stress incontinence, the patient should be examined in the Sim's position with a full bladder. The labia are parted, noting any excoriation, and the patient is asked to cough, and loss of urine and vaginal wall descent are noted. A Sim's speculum is inserted, and the anterior wall is observed again with coughing. Descent of the cervix is observed and traction may be applied using a sponge forceps holder on the anterior lip of the cervix. The speculum is gradually withdrawn noting any laxity of the posterior vaginal wall. A bimanual examination should be performed. The value of Bonney's test (elevation of the bladder neck) at the time of examination is debatable.

Investigations

MSU. Obviously it is important to rule out infection.

Urodynamic investigation. This should be performed in all cases of mixed symptoms, and debate exists as to whether it should be carried out in all cases.

Treatment

Local causes should be treated appropriately, e.g. infection.

Pelvic floor exercises, may be helpful, ideally under the guidance of a physiotherapist, and vaginal cones may be a useful adjunct.

Surgery is the mainstay of treatment and there are various options. Suprapubic operations are more effective for curing incontinence. The choice of operation depends on the degree of uterovaginal descent, and the general health of the patient.

1. Colposuspension. Sutures are placed periurethrally, and around the bladder neck, from above, and then sutured to the iliopectineal ligament, or the periosteum overlying the symphysis pubis.
2. Anterior colporrhaphy. The anterior wall of the vagina is elevated and any excess tissue is removed.
3. Sling procedures. These can be performed abdominally or vaginally, using synthetic material, or fascia lata to elevate the urethra. The sling is then attached to the rectus sheath.
4. Stamey procedures. A long needle is inserted abdominally and a suture is placed either side of the bladder neck to elevate it. The suture is secured to the rectus sheath. These procedures are becoming more popular.

Ring pessaries. If there is associated uterovaginal prolapse, these can be used in cases not fit for anaesthetic.

SUMMARY

Stress incontinence is a common problem which may be socially embarrassing and unhygienic. A careful history and examination is essential to make the correct diagnosis. Conservative treatment can be helpful but the definitive treatment is surgery, with suprapubic approaches giving better results.

URGE INCONTINENCE

Definition

Involuntary loss of urine caused by uninhibited detrusor contractions.

Interesting facts

Detrusor instability more commonly produces the classic triad of symptoms, namely, urgency, frequency, and nocturia (passing urine at night) without incontinence. It may be precipitated by a urinary tract infection, or gynaecological surgery.

Pathophysiology

In this condition the urethra functions normally but the bladder contracts in an uninhibited fashion, and if the intravesical pressure exceeds the urethral pressure, incontinence results.

Aetiology

1. Idiopathic
2. Secondary to an upper motor neurone lesion.

Assessment

History

History involves determining the severity of the following symptoms: frequency, urgency, and nocturia.

Examination

Examination is usually uninformative, but should include a full neurological examination.

Investigations

1. Microscopic examination of the urine.
2. Urodynamics: a normal bladder can be filled to at least 500 ml with an intravesical pressure rise of less than 10 cm of water. Normally, detrusor activity is suppressed with posture changes, sudden rises in intra-abdominal pressure and rapid filling. Cystometry measures intravesical pressure during bladder filling.
3. Detrusor instability is confirmed by a sensation of discomfort or a detrusor contraction (pressure rise > 15 cm water) during filling, coughing or standing.

Treatment

Bladder drill. This requires patient motivation for success. The aim is to progressively increase the interval between episodes of micturition. The usual interval should be determined, and the patient should then be instructed to pass urine at this frequency even if she has no desire to void. Once she has accomplished this, with no accidents, she should increase the time in 15-minute increments. This may take a few days, but once this is achieved, increase again, and again, until three hours is achieved. Essentially the bladder is 'retrained'. Ideally this should be done as an inpatient with biofeedback, but few units have these facilities.

Drug therapy

1. Anticholinergics. Currently the most popular of these agents is terodiline, which is a partial calcium antagonist. Anticholinergics are best used when bladder drill is initiated, and the patient can be weaned off the drug when control is achieved.
2. Ganglion blockers, e.g. emepronium bromide. These are out of favour at present as only 6% of the dose is absorbed and side-effects are unpleasant.
3. B-sympathomimetic agents, e.g. orciprenaline sulphate.
4. Oestrogen replacement.

Surgery. There is no place for surgery in the treatment of urge incontinence, and if attempted, it may worsen the situation.

Cystodistension. The bladder is distended to large volumes under anaesthesia, and although symptomatic relief may occur, studies have shown no objective improvement, and there is a 5% chance of bladder rupture.

SUMMARY

Detrusor instability produces the symptoms of urinary urgency, frequency, and nocturia. Cystometry is essential to confirm the diagnosis, and bladder drill ($\pm$ terodiline) is the treatment of choice.

OVERFLOW INCONTINENCE

Definition

Frequent involuntary loss of small volumes of urine, usually precipitated by changes in posture. The urinary stream is slow with hesitancy, and after micturition, there may be a sensation of incomplete emptying.

Pathophysiology

May be caused by obstruction to bladder outflow or bladder atony. Urine leakage occurs when the intravesical pressure exceeds the maximum urethral pressure in the absence of detrusor activity.

Aetiology

1. Upper or lower motor neurone lesions
2. Drugs, e.g. ganglion blockers, anticholinergic agents, B-adrenergic stimulants, tricyclic antidepressants
3. Surgery
4. Pelvic mass

5. Uterovaginal prolapse
6. Inflammation of the urethra, vulva, or vagina
7. Immobilization (especially in the elderly).

Assessment

History will provide the symptoms as above, and it may have been precipitated by a recent event. Examination may reveal a palpable mass. The passage of a urethral catheter will reveal a large residual urine.

Investigations

1. MSU
2. Cystometry will reveal a large residual urine with a delayed first sensation, and enlarged bladder capacity. The maximum voiding pressure will be normal or increased, and the peak flow rate will be slow.

Treatment

If drug ingestion is causing the problem, the drug regimen must be altered, and urine infection should be treated.

Pelvic masses and uterovaginal prolapse should be treated surgically. Ring pessaries may be helpful in correcting prolapse in the anaesthetically unfit patient.

Neurological causes are usually not treatable, and intermittent self-catheterization can be learnt.

SUMMARY

Overflow incontinence is not very satisfying to treat, but underlying pathology must be excluded.

TRUE INCONTINENCE

Definition

Continuous incontinence most commonly due to a fistulous track between the vagina and either the ureter, bladder, or urethra.

Interesting facts

Congenital abnormalities are rare, e.g. ureteric ectopy which presents in infancy.

A very low urethrovaginal fistula can cause intermittent incontinence.

Aetiology

1. Prolonged labour
2. Carcinoma
3. Surgery
4. Radiotherapy.

Assessment

History of urine continuously draining from the vagina. Examination is best performed in the Sim's position, with a Sim's speculum. Colouring the urine, and placing tampons in the vagina may aid location of the fistulous track.

Investigations

A micturating cystourethrogram, and/or an IVP may help location.

Treatment

1. Wait—some fistulae will heal spontaneously if given enough time with continuous bladder drainage.
2. Surgery.

FUNCTIONAL INCONTINENCE

Definition

Patient complains of intermittent or continuous incontinence but all investigations reveal no evidence of abnormality. Reassurance is helpful, and referral to a psychiatrist may be indicated.

B. Obstetrics

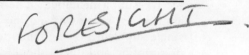

18. Prepregnancy counselling and prenatal diagnosis

G. Davis

PREPREGNANCY COUNSELLING

Expectations of the examiners

Candidates will be expected to know the range of disorders in which prepregnancy care is of benefit and the principles of management of the common conditions.

Definition

Prepregnancy counselling is the discussion and investigation of medical conditions either past or present which may influence fetal or maternal health in future pregnancies.

Interesting facts

Because of the emotional and financial cost of special care for infants or mothers with medical conditions, preventive medicine should be as widely practised as possible. Counselling is indicated in those women who are at risk of complications of medical illnesses that are evoked or worsened by pregnancy, or of giving birth to infants with genetic or environment related birth defects.

Assessment

An increasing number of women are seeking advice prior to pregnancy with questions concerning diet, smoking, alcohol, drugs and exercise. The use of multivitamins around the time of conception probably reduces the rate of recurrence of neural tube defects (NTDs) in at-risk women. In low-risk populations (South-east England) prophylaxis is not indicated. High-risk women (previous NTD, Northern Ireland) wishing to conceive should

143

receive supplementation. The active component of multivitamin preparations is unknown and no effects have been demonstrated using single supplements, e.g. zinc, folate. Smoking, alcohol, and drugs (both prescription and illicit) should be avoided. Prescription drugs should be reduced to minimal essential levels and changed to those known to be safe in early pregnancy if possible. There is no evidence that exercise adversely affects either conception or development (unless excessive exercise induces anovulation and amenorrhoea).

All these questions can be answered by the general practitioner but women with more specific problems as outlined in Table 18.1 should be referred to an obstetrician. Some of these problems can then be dealt with by the obstetrician directly, e.g. previous delivery experience, but others will require referral for further medical evaluation or genetic counselling. The obstetrician then remains the contact point for the woman, and can discuss with her the options given by physician or geneticist. Ideally, the woman should make an informed choice either to conceive, or rarely, to avoid conception.

Follow-up

It is essential that prepregnancy counselling is followed by consultation early in the pregnancy to confirm the presence of a viable intrauterine pregnancy, to allow accurate dating of the pregnancy and to arrange for prenatal diagnostic investigations if appropriate (see following section).

PRENATAL DIAGNOSIS OF FETAL ABNORMALITIES

Expectations of the examiners

Candidates will be expected to have a knowledge of the basic methods of prenatal diagnosis and the risks of common congenital disorders. They should also be familiar with the use and interpretation of routine prenatal screening tests for congenital anomalies.

Definition

Prenatal diagnosis is the detection of fetal disease or abnormality prior to delivery.

Interesting facts

Serious congenital abnormalities now account for 20% of perinatal deaths, are present in 2% of all births, and account for 30% of all paediatric admissions to hospital. Prenatal diagnosis is required in up to 10% of all

Table 18.1   Indications for prepregnancy counselling.

Maternal conditions
    Diabetes and other metabolic endocrine disorders
    Hypertension
    Specific maternal infections, e.g. genital herpes, HTLV III
    Risk of genetic disease, e.g. maternal age, family history of genetic abnormalities
    Drug exposure — either prescription or illicit
    Abnormal maternal nutrition, either obesity or subnormal weight
    Chronic medical problems, e.g. renal disease, SLE, heart disease, epilepsy,
    neurological disorders

Previous obstetric history
    Previous pregnancy loss, e.g. stillbirth, recurrent abortion
    Previous preterm delivery, growth retardation
    Previous infant with congenital anomaly or mental retardation
    Previous adverse delivery experience

pregnancies and although it has been described as 'preventive medicine', in reality many affected fetuses are terminated thereby removing them from the perinatal mortality statistics. However, some parents prefer to know if their child is abnormal prior to delivery in order to prepare themselves adequately for the birth.

Pathophysiology

Congenital abnormalities can be divided into four groups:

1. Chromosomal abnormalities arise during gamete formation or early in embryonic cleavage. They account for 40% of spontaneous abortions. Common examples are the trisomies 21 and 18, and Turner's syndrome 45XO. The incidence of all chromosomal disorders increases with age.
2. Single gene defects account for most of the inborn errors of metabolism.
3. Multifactorial influences usually result in structural abnormalities but some structural defects may occur in association with chromosomal abnormalities (e.g. duodenal atresia in Down syndrome) or drugs (e.g. phocomelia with thalidomide).
4. Environmental factors causing abnormality are mostly drugs or infections. Congenital infections may cause developmental abnormalities, intrauterine death or neonatal illness. Infections in this category include: rubella, syphilis, listeria, cytomegalovirus and toxoplasma.

Incidence of common congenital abnormalities

Down syndrome (trisomy 21)

Overall incidence 1 in 650 live births (LB). (See Table 18.2.)

Table 18.2 Incidence of Down syndrome.

Maternal age	Approximate risk of affected child	Risk of recurrence
20	1 in 2000	1 in 100
30	1 in 900	(irrespective of age)
35	1 in 365	
40	1 in 110	
42	1 in 70	
46	1 in 25	

Neural tube defects

The overall incidence of NTDs in the UK is difficult to determine as many affected fetuses abort or are terminated. The birth prevalence varies from 3.5–5 in 1000 total births in the North and West of the country to 2 in 1000 total births in the South and East. The recurrence rate is 1 in 20 after one affected child rising to 1 in 5 after 3 affected children. The risk of a NTD in the offspring of one affected parent is 5%, and 30% if both parents are affected. Fifty per cent of affected fetuses have anencephaly (which is incompatible with life), 45% spina bifida and 5% encephalocoeles. There are varying degrees of handicap but of those born with open spina bifida, 70% will die within the first five years and only 10% will be free of major handicap.

Congenital heart disease

The incidence of congenital heart disease is 8 per 1000 live births of which 50% are major defects. The recurrence risk is 1 in 50 and there is a 10% risk of having an affected child if one parent is affected.

Cystic fibrosis

Cystic fibrosis is inherited as a classical autosomal recessive trait with a birth prevalence of 1 per 2500. Males are sterile due to obliteration of the vas deferens but females can reproduce. The risk of an affected woman having an affected child is 1–2%.

Antenatal screening

Ninety per cent of congenital anomalies will arise in women who do not have any risk factors and screening is therefore important. Routine screening tests are:

1. Ultrasound at 16–18 weeks
2. Maternal AFP levels at 16 weeks
3. Testing for sickle cell disease in women of negroid extraction

4. Haemoglobin electrophoresis to detect thalassaemia in Mediterranean or Asian women
5. Testing for rubella immunity.

Routine anomaly scan

This is performed at 16–18 weeks to confirm the gestation and to exclude major fetal structural abnormalities. The fetus is carefully scanned with particular attention to the head, spine, four chamber view of the heart, kidneys, bowel, presence of a bladder and moving limbs of normal length. Ninety per cent of NTDs (the commonest structural abnormality) will be detected in this manner and it is rare to miss a major NTD.

Maternal serum alphafetoprotein (AFP) levels

These are raised in a large number of conditions, most commonly NTDs, but also in twin pregnancy, abdominal wall defects in the fetus, fetal death and fetal hydrops. Levels also rise as pregnancy progresses, therefore an accurate knowledge of gestation is essential for correct interpretation. Recently, low levels of maternal AFP have been shown to be associated with chromosomal abnormalities in the fetus.

Previously when the serum level was elevated the test was repeated, and if still high, amniocentesis performed. In many centres now, women with high AFP levels have a detailed ultrasound scan without repeating the test. If an abnormality is not detected, then karyotyping is performed. If a low AFP level is reported then the risk of Down syndrome is calculated and if it exceeds the risk for a woman of 35 years with normal AFP levels, then amniocentesis for karyotyping is performed.

Testing for sickle cell disease and thalassaemia

In women who have the disease or the trait, haemoglobin electrophoresis is performed on their partner's blood. If the partner is a carrier and hence the fetus at risk of having the disease, then direct testing of the fetal blood is required.

Rubella immunity

Most women are already immune to rubella through the nationwide immunization of teenage girls. Non-immune women are identified and managed appropriately.

Identification of risk groups

Women at risk of having a fetus with congenital abnormality are outlined in

Table 18.3 Women at risk of having a fetus with congenital abnormality.

History
  Previous abnormal child/fetus
  Family history of abnormality
  Maternal age > 35

Current pregnancy
  Maternal diabetes (4 × risk)
  Abnormal maternal AFP
  Exposure to teratogens — drugs, radiation
  Suspicious findings on routine ultrasound scan
  Breech presentation (4 × risk)
  Oligohydramnios
  Polyhydramnios
  Severe symmetrical growth retardation
  Twin pregnancy (2 × risk)
  Contact with or suspicion of maternal infection with known teratogenic pathogen,
  e.g. rubella, CMV

Table 18.3 and should be referred early in pregnancy for prenatal diagnosis.

Investigations

Methods

Ultrasound scan. This is used to detect structural abnormalities in the central nervous system, gastrointestinal tract, urinary system, skeleton and heart. In addition, cleft lip and palate can be detected if a specific search is made. Routine ultrasound screening for structural abnormalities is performed at 16–18 weeks which is a compromise between performing the procedure earlier (so that safer termination of pregnancy may be carried out) and later (when the structural details become more obvious).

Amniocentesis. Removal of liquor for the culture of desquamated fetal fibroblasts permits karyotyping and the detection of enzyme defects. This is now performed under ultrasound guidance. It takes 2–3 weeks for the cells to proliferate sufficiently for investigation and culture is unsuccessful in < 5% of cases. It is ideally performed between 16–18 weeks when sufficient liquor is available, although recently several groups have reported its successful use at 12–14 weeks. The risk of the procedure to the pregnancy is 1% greater than the 1% risk of fetal loss at 16 weeks (total 2%).

Chorion villus biopsy (CVS). CVS involves aspirating placental tissue under ultrasound guidance either transcervically or transabdominally with a needle. Karyotyping and other investigations can usually be performed immediately on placental tissue, significantly reducing the delay between the procedure and result. It is also carried out earlier in pregnancy (9–12 weeks) permitting earlier, safer termination if necessary. Fetal losses due to the procedure are reported to be 2% but probably improve as the operator gains experience.

Cordocentesis. Ultrasound guided sampling from the umbilical cord permits the direct assessment of the fetal blood, e.g. acid-base status, haemoglobinopathies, electrolytes and pathogens and is possible after 18 weeks' gestation. Because of the invasive nature of this technique, its use is restricted to at-risk fetuses, e.g. severe growth retardation, suspected congenital infection and structural cardiac abnormality, and it is now used routinely for intrauterine transfusions of fetuses with haemolytic disease. Rates of fetal loss are not high but figures are difficult to obtain because of the high-risk group in which the procedure is used.

Fetoscopy. An alternative method for sampling fetal blood or tissue is to do so under direct vision using a fine laparoscope. Fetal losses from this procedure are reported to be about 3% but the technique has been largely superseded by cordocentesis.

Magnetic resonance imaging. This is the most recently developed tool used in the diagnosis of fetal abnormalities and its place has yet to be determined.

Laboratory investigations

Chromosome analysis. Nuclei are either stained immediately (chorion villus biopsy, cordocentesis) or the cells are cultured and then the nuclei are stained. Duplication of chromosomes and gross rearrangements (e.g. translocations) are then detectable. The commonest chromosomal abnormalities which survive until term are the trisomies (21, 18, 13) and Turner's syndrome (45XO).

Enzyme defects. These are usually detected by direct assay in chorionic villi or occasionally by incubation of fetal cells with a specific substrate. It is only possible where the fetus is known to be at risk of an inborn error of metabolism, i.e. where the parents have had an affected infant previously or screening has revealed the parents to be carriers.

Tests on fetal blood. A number of haematological parameters may be measured directly on fetal blood, e.g. factor VIII to detect haemophilia A and beta globin to detect thalassemia. These methods are largely being replaced by gene probe analysis (see below). Recently, fetal blood sampling to assess acid-base status and electrolytes has become more common in high-risk pregnancies. This is currently only of value after fetal viability (24 weeks' gestation) and is used to assist in the management of severely compromised fetuses. As experience in this field increases, its use will undoubtedly increase.

DNA probe analysis. Using these methods, abnormal genes are detected in two ways, either directly or indirectly (linkage studies). Direct detection is possible where the specific mutation has been identified, e.g sickle cell disease or cystic fibrosis. Indirect detection relies on the fact that

Table 18.4   Conditions for which probes are available.

X linked recessive
  Duchenne muscular dystrophy
  Fragile X syndrome
  Haemophilia A and B

Autosomal recessive
  Cystic fibrosis
  Phenylketonuria
  Sickle cell anaemia
  Thalassemia

Autosomal dominant
  Huntington's chorea
  Neurofibromatosis

most chromosomes have differences in the DNA sequence of homologous (same number, e.g. 21) chromosomes which do not cause genetic disease (polymorphism). If a mutation is close to a *detectable* polymorphic change, then the mutation and the polymorphic change will usually travel together in any recombination of genetic material that occurs. In this way, the polymorphic marker can be used to determine whether the fetus has the affected gene.

Some of the more common conditions for which gene probes are now available are listed in Table 18.4.

Management of at-risk couples

Irrespective of whether at-risk couples opt for termination of pregnancy or not, genetic counselling is of value. General practitioners and obstetricians should be familiar with the risks and preliminary management of the conditions for which women are routinely screened in antenatal clinics. For at-risk couples, most practitioners will need to involve a medical geneticist, although the management principles are the same.

These principles include:

1. Knowledge of which couples are at risk from their history or clinical features. It is important that the diagnosis of the affected member(s) of the family is accurate before proceeding further
2. The natural history of the disease
3. The range of its clinical manifestations
4. Possibility of treatment, and risks of treatment
5. Accuracy of treatment and prognosis
6. Possibility of detecting carriers
7. Psychological implications
8. Likelihood of recurrence and management in subsequent pregnancy.

It is important that information, which is often quite complex, is presented to the parents in a way which they can understand. Although it is impossible to present information in an unbiased manner, this should be the goal. Genetic counselling has been shown to fail to educate at-risk couples adequately in 40% of cases, so repeated counselling is usually necessary. Other attendants involved in their care should avoid confusing the situation if they are not fully conversant with the disorder. Couples will often experience grief which must be dealt with before information can be passed on. Most couples then regard the problem in terms of how it will affect their relationship, their immediate family and their financial status.

Follow-up

The need for close follow-up of affected pregnancies is self evident. If an affected child is delivered, then ongoing paediatric care is usually necessary and the couple then need to return for reinforcement of the information on outcome of the affected child and recurrence risk in future children. Couples that have opted for termination of pregnancy attend for the results of the post mortem (if possible) and to discuss again the possibility of, and management in, subsequent pregnancy.

19. Antenatal care

G. Davis

Expectations of the examiners

The routine management of pregnancy and the assessment of obstetric risk are fundamental to the appropriate care of obstetric patients and the examiners will therefore expect candidates to have a comprehensive grasp of all aspects.

Definition

'A planned programme of observation, education, and medical management of pregnant women directed toward making pregnancy and delivery a safe and satisfying experience.' *American College of Obstetricians and Gynaecologists.*

Interesting facts

The major objective of antenatal care is to reduce perinatal and maternal morbidity and mortality. Whether this objective is best achieved by the manner in which antenatal care is currently practised is debatable. At least 80% of pregnant women would deliver healthy babies without any antenatal care and very few of the measures used routinely have been properly evaluated.

The objectives of antenatal care are:

1. To predict problems on the basis of the medical, social and obstetric history and physical examination of the women.
2. To prevent, or reduce the severity of problems by prophylactic measures.
3. To detect and treat conditions which have harmful effects on mother or fetus.
4. To provide education, information and reassurance for the pregnant woman and her partner.

The current approach to routine antenatal care ideally involves:

1. Prepregnancy counselling (see Ch. 18)

2. Booking visit
3. Routine antenatal visits
4. Antenatal education classes
5. Inpatient care if required.

BOOKING VISIT

Assessment

The booking visit is the most important visit in most women's antenatal care. At this visit, risk factors are assessed and future antenatal care and place of delivery decided. Pregnant women are usually seen by a midwife initially and a history taken, special investigations performed or ordered, information on maternity benefits and antenatal education classes given and a date made for a further appointment. At the next visit the woman sees a member of the medical staff, by which time results of initial investigations are available to assist in further decisions. This process may also be completed at a single visit.

Timing

Ideally the woman should be seen as early as possible to confirm pregnancy and to deal with any early problems, e.g. chorion villus biopsy at 8–12 weeks. At the latest, the woman should be seen at 16–18 weeks' gestation to allow maternal alpha fetoprotein determination, assessment of gestational age and exclusion of structural anomalies by ultrasound, and amniocentesis if necessary.

History

The booking history should include:

1. Identification details
2. Social history
3. Menstrual/contraceptive history
4. Medical conditions
5. Past obstetric history
6. Factors associated with genetic risk
7. General condition.

Identification details. These should include the woman's full name, address, next of kin, and race. In addition, her general practitioner's name, address and whether he or she wishes to undertake shared care should be recorded.

Social history. Details of the woman's occupation, marital status and social circumstances should be noted. It should include her attitude to the pregnancy and that of her partner. Her partner's race, occupation and support should be recorded. Details of housing are important as these may need to be changed during pregnancy and eligibility for benefits assessed.

A full drug history should be obtained including prescribed and illicit drugs, alcohol and tobacco. All women should be encouraged to give up the latter three and prescribed medications may need to be modified in pregnancy.

Menstrual/contraceptive history. The date (and degree of certainty) of the last menstrual period (LMP) must be established and the regularity and length of the menstrual cycle. If the LMP was abnormal the last normal menstrual period should be recorded and any subsequent bleeding. If the woman was using the combined oral contraceptive then it should be determined whether the LMP was a withdrawal bleed. In some cases, such as pregnancy after a period of amenorrhoea or after previous pregnancy, no menstrual history is available. Previous duration and treatment of infertility should be noted.

If an intrauterine device is still present (and the strings are visible on examination) this should be removed to reduce the possibility of later septic abortions. As in all women of reproductive age who present with amenorrhoea, ectopic pregnancy should be excluded.

Past obstetric history. This is the most important part of the history in terms of identifying risk factors in the current pregnancy. Details of all previous pregnancies including abortions, terminations of pregnancy and ectopic pregnancies should be recorded. The gestations of previous pregnancies, complications and details of delivery and postnatal complications should be noted. The paternity of all previous pregnancies should also be determined. Previous stillbirth or intrauterine growth retardation is an indication for increased monitoring of fetal well-being in the third trimester. A history of recurrent, painless mid-trimester abortion suggests cervical incompetence which may require a cervical suture. A previous baby delivered spontaneously and prematurely is the best predictor of preterm delivery in the current pregnancy. If a previous baby was delivered by caesarean section, the indications for operation, type of procedure and woman's attitude to the operation must be carefully determined to assess whether a trial of labour is suitable. This may require communication with a previous hospital. Any problems in the third stage of labour will necessitate the presence of an obstetrician at subsequent deliveries. A previous baby with a congenital abnormality or other neonatal problems may be an indication for prenatal diagnosis.

Medical conditions. Any medical condition in the woman should be noted. A brief series of direct questions to exclude major disease should include:

1. Diabetes mellitus (pregnancy induced or otherwise)
2. Epilepsy

3. Thromboembolic disease
4. Anaemia
5. Chest diseases
6. Tuberculosis
7. Hypertension
8. Cardiac disease (congenital or acquired)
9. Renal disease
10. Endocrine disease (thyroid, adrenal)
11. Sexually transmitted disease
12. Rubella.

All of these conditions affect, or are affected by, pregnancy to a greater or lesser extent.

Previous operations, particularly those with relevance to the pregnancy, e.g. previous cone biopsy (risk of cervical incompetence) or bladder surgery (risk of weakening repair) should be recorded. Any psychiatric history increases the risk of postpartum psychiatric problems and should be specifically elicited as many women wish to avoid discussing this. Any allergies should be prominently recorded in the hospital notes and any record the woman keeps.

All women should be asked the date and result of their last cervical smear and this should be repeated if it has not been done in the previous three years or was previously abnormal.

Genetic risk. Individuals at increased risk of fetal abnormality include:

1. Maternal age greater than 35 years—risk of chromosomal abnormality
2. Negroid women—risk of sickle cell disease
3. Mediterranean or Asian women—risk of thalassaemia
4. Ashkenazi Jews—risk of Tay–Sachs disease
5. Previous child with abnormality
6. Family history of fetal abnormality, inherited diseases, e.g. haemophilia.

Prenatal diagnosis should be discussed with all these women and appropriate action taken (see Ch. 18).

General condition. The woman should be asked if she has any complaints currently including vaginal bleeding or discharge, vomiting or concern over the pregnancy. Any questions the woman has about antenatal care or her health should be answered at this stage.

Examination

The woman should be weighed and her height and blood pressure measured. The cardiovascular and respiratory systems are examined and the breasts checked for masses or inverted nipples. Abdominal examination is performed to confirm the presence of a pelvic mass (after 12 weeks' gestation) or later in pregnancy, fetal growth, presentation and lie.

The fundus reaches the umbilicus at 20–24 weeks' gestation and the xiphisternum at 36–38 weeks. The presence of the fetal heart is confirmed with a Pinard fetal stethoscope (after 32 weeks' gestation) or a sonicaid (after 12–14 weeks). The lie is readily determined after 28–30 weeks.

Pelvic examination confirms gestation, excludes pelvic pathology and permits a cervical smear to be taken. However, unless a cervical smear is required, the value of a routine pelvic examination is debatable in a setting where routine ultrasound is performed.

Investigations

Blood tests

The blood tests routinely performed at booking are:

1. FBC
2. Blood group and antibody screen
3. Hepatitis serology
4. Syphilis serology
5. Rubella serology.

Also in at-risk groups:

1. Sickle test
2. Haemoglobin electrophoresis.

The most common form of anaemia detected is due to iron deficiency. The lower limit of normal in pregnancy is reduced because of the haemo-dilution that occurs (10.5 or 11 g/dl). If the hepatitis serology is positive (HBsAg) then further testing for HBeAg and HBsAb is carried out. Routine testing for syphilis usually includes VDRL and TPHA and if positive, testing for current infection is carried out. Rubella immunity is assessed by screening for IgG unless there has been a possible recent contact, in which case the IgM levels are measured and repeated in two weeks to look for a rise in titre (indicating recent infection). If the IgG is negative and there is no prenatal infection, vaccination is performed after delivery.

Maternal serum alpha fetoprotein (AFP)

This is measured at 16–18 weeks and if it is more than 2.5 times the mean for gestation, further testing is required to exclude neural tube defects or other abnormality. Low AFP levels are associated with Down syndrome (see Ch. 18).

Routine ultrasound scan

In most units this is carried out at 16–18 weeks for the following reasons:

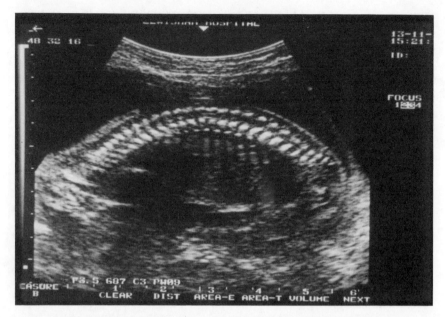

Fig. 19.1   Ultrasound scan in which the spine is seen in its entirety.

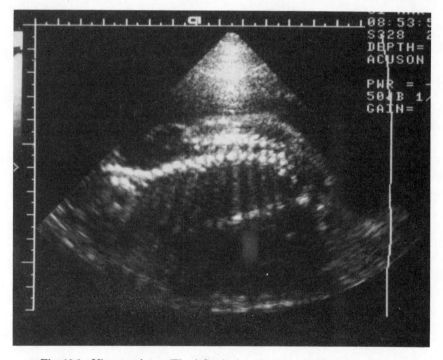

Fig. 19.2   Ultrasound scan. The defect in the spine (spina bifida) is clearly seen.

1. Accurate assessment of gestation—even in those women with certain dates, ultrasound has been demonstrated to be more accurate. It is also important for optimal interpretation of maternal serum alpha fetoprotein levels.
2. Detection of multiple pregnancy.
3. Detection of congenital abnormalities in the fetus.
4. Baseline for further scans if necessary later in the pregnancy.
5. Determination of the placental site. Although the placental site can usually be detected accurately at this gestation, many units do not routinely rescan those women with a low lying placenta because the vast majority will resolve as the lower segment forms at 28–34 weeks.
6. Reassurance for mother and partner.

There has never been any reliable evidence that ultrasound used as it is in the prenatal period is dangerous for the fetus (or the mother).

Assessment of risk

Many lists of risk factors have been published and a recent one is included in the Appendix. Failing to identify risk factors or to take appropriate action when they are known to be present is a common error in obstetric practice. Obstetric patients can be classified as having low, moderate or high risk and their pregnancy managed accordingly. Risk based on factors in the history is assessed at the booking visit but the development of any problems in pregnancy may necessitate a reappraisal of the degree of risk.

Type of antenatal care

For most women this will be a choice between full hospital care or care shared between general practitioner and hospital. For low-risk patients, shared care is usually more convenient and reduces waiting times in hospital antenatal clinics. High risk patients should usually be seen exclusively at the hospital while the care of those with moderate risk should be decided individually.

Place of delivery

Only 1% of women now deliver at home. If the woman wishes to do so, then she must be at low risk and be supervized by a registered domiciliary midwife and doctor. Ideally, these women should be seen at the hospital for a booking visit and at least one visit later in pregnancy although, in practice, some women who opt for home delivery avoid hospitals. Low-risk patients suitable for home delivery must:

1. Be healthy women aged 19 to 34 years

2. Be para one or two
3. Have no major contraindications.

Major contraindications include:

1. Previous complicated obstetric/medical history
2. Major gynaecological surgery or condition (including infertility)
3. Under 152 cm in height (5 ft)
4. Gross obesity
5. Any abnormality in current pregnancy
6. Postmaturity in current pregnancy
7. Severe social problems
8. No phone available/difficult access.

An alternative to home delivery offered in most delivery units is 'domino' (domiciliary in and out) care. Women in labour of low or moderate risk are cared for in the delivery unit by domiciliary midwives and, provided all is normal, discharged 6–12 hours after delivery. If there are any problems in labour, then care can be safely and efficiently transferred to the hospital.

SUBSEQUENT VISITS

The timing of routine antenatal visits is variable but is usually every four weeks until 28 weeks, fortnightly until 36 weeks and weekly thereafter. If the woman is receiving shared care then the same routine should be followed but hospital visits should be at 32 weeks, and weekly from 39 or 40 weeks.

There is wide variation between hospitals on the timing of these visits. If an abnormality is detected then the frequency of visits is increased and care may be transferred completely to the hospital.

Examination

As most antenatal visits will reveal no abnormality, it is important to avoid complacency and to maintain a high degree of alertness to potential problems. At each visit, the woman's weight and sitting blood pressure are measured and a urine sample tested for protein and glucose. More than average weight gain may be associated with fluid retention as a result of pre-eclampsia.

The blood pressure usually falls in the second trimester and should be considered abnormal if it is more than 140/90 on two separate occasions 24 hours apart, or if there is a rise of 20 mmHg or greater in the diastolic pressure.

Proteinuria may be due to contamination of the specimen by vaginal discharge. If present on a mid-stream urine early in pregnancy, it is usually due to infection or chronic renal disease and these should be investigated appropriately. Its appearance later in pregnancy suggests infection again or serious pre-eclampsia and in the presence of even mildly elevated blood pressure warrants admission for further assessment.

Glycosuria on more than one occasion is an indication for an oral glucose tolerance test to exclude maternal diabetes although it is commonly due to the lowered renal threshold for glucose excretion in pregnancy.

Abdominal examination is performed to assess fetal growth and the symphysiofundal height may be measured. There is considerable debate over the relative merits of the tape measure vs. the hand but candidates should be able to use a tape measure to assess fundal height whatever their clinical practice. The most important diagnostic aid is a high degree of awareness. The liquor volume is assessed and presentation checked from 32 weeks. After 36 weeks persistent breech presentation should be managed appropriately (see Ch. 28). The fetal head usually engages from 36–38 weeks in nulliparous women but in at least 40% of parous women, engagement does not occur until labour begins. An unengaged head may be due to:

1. Pelvic mass—placenta praevia, tumour
2. Large presenting diameter—hydrocephalus, malpresentation, malposition
3. Large uterus—polyhydramnios, multiple pregnancy
4. Small pelvis—cephalopelvic disproportion, abnormal pelvis.

The ease with which the head enters the pelvis can be determined by gently pressing the head into the pelvis with the woman semi-seated. A pelvic examination should be performed to exclude major bony abnormality, and many obstetricians will repeat the ultrasound scan if the head remains high after 38 weeks.

Investigations

Routine screening tests have been described. The haemoglobin concentration and antibody titres in rhesus-negative women are measured at 30 and 36 weeks unless they are abnormal.

The most common causes of anaemia in pregnancy are iron deficiency, and folate deficiency. These can be almost completely avoided by the administration of combined iron/folate preparations but many women find them difficult to take. Opinion on their routine use varies, but anaemia, particularly if associated with microcytosis and/or hypochromasia, should be treated with oral iron. Women should be seen weekly and compliance checked by asking the woman the colour of her stools, and measuring the haemoglobin concentration and reticulocyte count. Iron infusion is dangerous and it is better to admit the woman to ensure compliance rather than give an iron infusion.

In many centres, rhesus-negative women are routinely given anti-D gammaglobulin at 28 and 34 weeks to reduce the incidence of sensitization prior to delivery.

Assessment of fetal growth and/or well-being

One of the major reasons for antenatal care is the detection of reduced fetal growth and yet failure to do so is common (50% undetected). The means of monitoring fetal well-being/growth are:

1. Clinical assessment at antenatal visits
2. Fetal movements
3. Ultrasound assessment
4. Biophysical profile on the fetus
5. Fetal heart rate recordings
6. Fetoplacental blood flow
7. Cordocentesis.

The use of tests of placental synthetic function, e.g. urinary oestriol, HPL, has largely been superseded by other measures. This is principally because these tests do not specifically measure fetal well-being and may be affected by a number of factors, e.g. technical aspects of measuring levels, antibiotic therapy, individual variation.

Clinical assessment

The importance of vigilance during routine antenatal clinics has been stressed.

Fetal movements

Every pregnant woman attending for antenatal care should be questioned regarding fetal movements over the preceding few days. A significant decrease in movements warrants further investigation, i.e. ultrasound scan and fetal heart rate recording and subsequent closer surveillance.

Most women report that their babies move less towards term and it often remains difficult to assess. It is better to be overcautious in this respect. The efficacy of fetal movement charts is debated but they probably make women more aware of fetal activity.

Ultrasound assessment

Ultrasound will only assess fetal growth if used in a serial manner. Although a single scan may suggest growth retardation, i.e. disproportionately low overall fetal measurements (symmetrical growth retardation), or reduced abdominal circumference (asymmetrical growth retardation) or reduced liquor volume, a follow-up scan is often necessary to assess growth. The routine scan at 16–18 weeks is vital to confirm that gestation is correct.

Biophysical profile

A fetal heart rate monitor and ultrasound machine are used simultaneously to assess in the fetus:

1. Breathing movements
2. Limb and body movements
3. Tone
4. Heart rate
5. Amniotic fluid volume.

   Each of these variables is scored to make up the profile. Their use in routine obstetric practice is still being evaluated, the problem being that they are time-consuming and there is wide variation in these variables in healthy fetuses.

Fetal heart rate recording

This gives an indication of the current status of the fetus. A normal pattern with accelerations in response to fetal movements is a good indication of fetal well-being.

   The significance of other patterns is difficult to interpret, particularly in very preterm fetuses. The presence of decelerations when the woman is not in labour usually indicates that immediate delivery is required.

Fetoplacental blood flow

The use of the Doppler principle to measure blood flow in the uterine and umbilical vessels and the fetal arterial system is a recent innovation. Studies on the use of Doppler as a screening test for detecting fetal compromise to date have shown no clear benefit. Its use at present is restricted to being part of the assessment of fetuses already known to be compromised.

   Reduced, absent, or even retrograde flow in the umbilical artery during diastole is an indication of increased placental resistance and therefore probably impaired fetal oxygenation. Used in conjunction with other tests it may help in making the decision on when to deliver preterm fetuses.

Cordocentesis

Cordocentesis is now being used to monitor the condition of the severely compromised fetus. This usually means severe growth retardation at 24–30 weeks' gestation or significant fetal structural abnormality. The measurement of fetal arterial pH, acid-base status and oxygenation is now being used in the management of these difficult problems in specialized units.

General advice in pregnancy

Pregnancy is a stressful time for both partners (and other children). Antenatal visits should provide the opportunity for women to ask about minor problems as well as ensuring that all screening tests and routine assessment is carried out. Most hospital clinics provide mothers with an easily readable information booklet, e.g. *Pregnancy Book* by the Health Education Council.

Diet

Although pregnancy increases the mother's dietary requirements, a balanced diet is sufficient to provide all the calories, protein, minerals and vitamins required. The only exception is iron. If iron is not given in pregnancy, iron stores will decline. However, provided that these were adequate initially this is not a problem. Women who are already anaemic, have depleted iron stores (grand multipara, recent pregnancy) or who have a multiple pregnancy should have combined iron and folate supplementation.

Exercise

The amount of exercise desirable in pregnancy has never been determined. It seems prudent not to begin vigorous exercise when pregnant and similarly safe to continue routine exercise as long as it is not causing serious discomfort.

Sexual activity

There is no evidence that coitus is harmful in pregnancy. Most obstetricians advise against coitus in the first trimester in women who have had recurrent abortions, but there is no evidence to support this view.

Many women lose their inclination for sex as pregnancy advances because of their increasing awkwardness and feelings of not being attractive. Couples should be encouraged to communicate these feelings. Sexual techniques may need to be modified to avoid pressure on the uterus.

Rest and sleep

Most women are more easily fatigued in pregnancy and there is some evidence that regular resting improves fetal outcome. Resting should therefore be encouraged, particularly in women with demanding lives.

Sleep patterns tend to become less regular with more frequent waking as pregnancy continues and women may need daytime naps to catch up.

Employment

The evidence on the effect of work on pregnancy is difficult to assess. Jobs involving a lot of standing may lead to reduced fetal growth but other variables are important, such as the number of children the pregnant woman cares for at home. It seems sensible to advise each woman individually depending on her wishes, type of work and demands of her home life.

Heavy manual labour should be avoided and pregnant women must be allowed to rest if necessary. Noxious fumes, extremes of temperature and working to exhaustion should be avoided.

Clothing

A supportive brassiere and comfortable clothes are the basic requirements. Most women find flat-heeled shoes more comfortable in later pregnancy.

Preparation for lactation

All participants in antenatal care should strongly encourage breast-feeding. In the antenatal period it is important to ensure that the woman understands the advantages of breast-feeding and the normal events in milk production after delivery.

There is no need to encourage frequent handling of the nipples to prepare them for feeding. Inverted nipples usually correct themselves during pregnancy and can be made to protrude with gentle manipulation. If these measures are unsuccessful then nipple shields are used and kept in place by the brassiere.

Antenatal education

Classes are usually available in hospital clinics. A wide range of matters need to be covered including changes in late pregnancy, when to come in to delivery suite, choice of methods for delivery position and pain relief, what clothes the baby will need and when to buy them, how to cope with a new baby and discussion on how the baby is likely to affect the couple.

Most classes take prospective parents on a tour of the labour and postnatal wards to prepare them for delivery. Birth plans are encouraged at most hospitals but it is important to emphasize that labour and delivery can be unpredictable and that all women (and their partners) need to retain an open mind. Questioning should be encouraged and all answers should be given in terms which can be easily understood.

Follow-up

One of the most important aspects of antenatal care is that follow-up should occur so that the woman and her partner have the opportunity to discuss their labour and management. Much of this discussion occurs on the postnatal ward and with the visits of the domiciliary midwife after discharge from hospital. This information is important in ensuring that misunderstandings are corrected and negative experiences discussed.

20. Minor disorders of pregnancy

G. Davis

Expectations of the examiners

As these disorders are not usually disabling they are often treated initially by general practitioners. The examiners will therefore expect candidates to have a sound knowledge of their causes and a common sense approach to their management.

Nausea and vomiting

The majority of women experience some nausea in early pregnancy and 50% will vomit. Although classically worse in the mornings it may occur throughout the day and is often made worse by the odours associated with preparing food. If severe, multiple pregnancy and hydatidiform mole need to be excluded. Symptoms usually improve after 14–16 weeks although many women continue to experience nausea, and sometimes vomiting, more frequently than when not pregnant.

Management

In most instances, symptoms can be controlled by dietary measures. Greasy or highly-spiced foods should be avoided and frequent small meals usually improve the nausea. A rearrangement of housekeeping duties may be required if the woman is responsible for these. Reassurance, practical help in coping with the symptoms and the knowledge that the problem usually improves, are important aspects of the medical care.

Admission to hospital is required if the woman is becoming dehydrated (ketones in urine), if there is significant weight loss or if the social situation is getting out of control. In hospital, fluids are given intravenously (with potassium supplementation), antiemetics are used (initially metoclopramide then prochlorperazine if this is ineffective) and no oral intake is permitted. The condition is usually improving by 24–36 hours and dry biscuits can usually be introduced by 48 hours. If there is no improvement, then intravenous alimentation may be required. Early discharge from hospital is discouraged as it is often followed by prompt readmission.

Heartburn

This is also common in pregnancy and results from gastric reflux due to relaxation of the lower oesophageal sphincter and pressure from the enlarging uterus later in pregnancy.

The condition should be treated by discouraging smoking (increases sphincter relaxation), recommending frequent, light, bland meals and avoiding a late meal, and raising the head of the bed about 20 cm. Antacid preparations, e.g. magnesium trisilicate may also be helpful but those that are likely to cause constipation should be avoided (aluminium containing).

Constipation/bloating

It is thought that these symptoms are due to decreased bowel motility because of high levels of progesterone. Normal measures should be used to combat constipation: dietary fibre and fluid intake should increase, sugar intake should decrease and a bulk laxative, e.g. ispaghula husk, used if necessary. Bloating seems to occur independently and is difficult to treat effectively.

Haemorrhoids

These occur more frequently in pregnancy due to progesterone-induced venodilatation, obstruction of venous return from the lower body by the enlarged uterus, and increased bearing down because of constipation or at delivery.

Prolapse is best treated with ice packs and replacement if possible. Bleeding is common and a rectal examination should be performed in this instance. For mild symptoms, a soothing preparation with a mild astringent action is usually sufficient. Rarely surgical intervention may be necessary.

Epistaxis

This occurs as a result of increased peripheral vascularity. Normal first aid measures usually suffice and definitive treatment is rarely necessary.

Varicose veins

Varicosities occur mostly in the legs but also in the vulva and vagina and cause aching and tiredness. Thrombophlebitis is the commonest complication and deep venous thrombosis may also occur although this is more common in the puerperium.

For leg varicosities, the best treatment is a combination of elevation and the use of full-length support tights. Surgical management is best reserved for at least 2–3 months postpartum when the veins will have returned to normal after pregnancy.

Backache

This is a common symptom and results from increased joint laxity in the lumbar spine and the exaggerated lordosis which occurs in pregnancy. Sacroiliac joint laxity may also cause pain. Management is conservative: rest, analgesia and improvement in posture.

Breast soreness

This is commonest in early pregnancy as the breasts increase in size. Reassurance and symptomatic relief with a brassiere that provides adequate support are all that is needed.

Fatigue

This is a common symptom early in pregnancy when the cause is unclear, and late in pregnancy when it is due to the increased physical effort required for everyday life and often a disturbed sleep pattern. The only treatment is frequent rest and reassurance that it is normal.

Peripheral paraesthesia

Numbness and tingling occur due to compression of peripheral nerves because of fluid retention, most commonly the median nerve (carpal tunnel syndrome). Other nerves may be affected such as the lateral cutaneous nerve of the thigh which supplies the lateral aspect of the thigh. No treatment is usually required when the cause has been explained to the patient.

Headache

This is usually a typical tension headache and is best treated by rest and mild analgesia. Migraine often improves but may deteriorate, stay the same or occur de novo, in pregnancy. The use in pregnancy of agents normally used in the treatment of migraine is not associated with adverse fetal outcome but doses should be kept to the minimum required.

Postural hypotension

This is more likely to occur in pregnancy because of venous pooling in the lower limbs (see Haemorrhoids above). It is best prevented by avoiding precipitating factors: standing up quickly, hot baths, standing in hot weather.

Pruritus

Itching in pregnancy may be localized or generalized. Local causes are usually infectious (e.g. scabies, thrush). Generalized itching (pruritus gravidarum) usually begins in the third trimester and is almost always associated with some degree of biliary obstruction. Frank jaundice is rare but cholestasis of pregnancy must be distinguished from other causes of liver disease in pregnancy and non-pregnancy.

Fetal outcome is not affected except in those women developing clinical jaundice. The pruritus disappears shortly after delivery but recurs in 50% of subsequent pregnancies. Treatment with skin lubrication and topical antipruritics is usually sufficient and antihistamines are of limited benefit.

Frequency of micturition

Again this is a symptom of early pregnancy when it may be due to increased renal filtration, and of late pregnancy when it is due to pressure from the enlarged uterus. There is no treatment for this symptom except delivery. Urinary tract infection is also common in pregnancy and needs to be excluded.

Insomnia

Disturbed sleep results from normal anxieties about being pregnant and later the increased size of breasts and abdomen. Sedatives should be avoided unless the woman is exhausted and should then be used for a very brief period, e.g. 2–3 nights. Relaxation exercises to relieve anxiety may be of benefit.

SUMMARY

Minor disorders of pregnancy are very common but serious conditions need to be excluded, e.g. imminent eclampsia causing headache, viral hepatitis causing pruritus. Education and reassurance together with simple, practical remedies are the basis for treatment of most of these conditions.

21. Infections in pregnancy

A. Rodin

Expectations of the examiners

An understanding of the effects on the mother and the fetus of significant infections in pregnancy is needed.

Interesting facts

Maternal infections during pregnancy are common and are usually insignificant but may result in congenital infection and handicap. The incidence of death or handicap as a result of intrauterine infection is estimated to be 0.4 in 1000 live births. The incidence of many congenital infections shows marked regional variation, for example, toxoplasmosis is commoner in France than in the UK. In some cases, congenital infections can be prevented and/or treated.

Pathogenesis

Infections may reach the fetus by four main routes:

1. Transplacental spread from the maternal bloodstream
2. Ascending infection from the genital tract after rupture of membranes
3. Infection acquired during passage of the fetus through the birth canal
4. Rarely, infection may follow invasive intra-amniotic procedures, e.g. amniocentesis and fetoscopy.

The effects on the fetus depend on the nature of the infective organism, the gestation at which infection occurs and the immune status of the mother.

Following maternal infection there may be no spread to the fetus, however it may reach the placenta and infect the fetus in utero. Fetal infection may manifest itself by abortion or stillbirth. If the pregnancy continues, the infant may be born with a variety of abnormalities (TORCH syndrome—see below) and it may develop acute neonatal illness. An infant of an infected mother who appears normal at birth may develop late effects and should be followed up.

The infectious agents causing the TORCH syndrome are:

1. Toxoplasmosis
2. Rubella
3. Cytomegalovirus
4. Herpes simplex.

These cause a mild, non-specific maternal illness and similar patterns of fetal damage. Features of the TORCH syndrome include:

1. Low birth weight
2. Microcephaly
3. Congenital heart disease
4. Eye lesions
5. Jaundice
6. Hepatosplenomegaly
7. Petechiae/purpura
8. Late effects:
    a. Visual defects
    b. Deafness
    c. Developmental delay
    d. Mental retardation.

RUBELLA

The association between maternal rubella infection in pregnancy and congenital heart disease and cataracts in the neonate was first described in 1941. Rubella is a RNA virus and is spread by droplet infection.

Maternal illness

Mild febrile illness with a macular rash and lymphadenopathy; many infections are subclinical. One infection confers a high degree of immunity and congenital infection only follows primary maternal infection.

Fetal effects

The risk of congenital defects depends on the gestation when infection occurs: infection in the first trimester carries a high risk of major defects and infection between 12 to 16 weeks may cause sensorineural deafness.

Hearing impairment is the most frequent defect associated with rubella.

Screening

All women are screened for rubella antibody (IgG) at booking. Susceptible women who develop a rash or come into contact with rubella have blood taken to check rubella IgG. If this is positive, IgM is measured to confirm recent infection.

Immunization

A live attenuated virus vaccine was introduced in 1970 and this was given to prepubertal girls and non-immune women.

Ninety-eight per cent of women in the UK attending antenatal clinics are now immune to rubella.

In 1988, the MMR vaccination (measles, mumps and rubella) was introduced and this is given to all male and female infants between 1–2 years of age in an attempt to eradicate rubella. Vaccination of prepubertal girls and non-immune women will continue until sufficient numbers have received MMR vaccination.

Vaccination should not be administered during pregnancy and conception within three months should be avoided.

CYTOMEGALOVIRUS

Cytomegalovirus (CMV) is the most common congenital infection and approximately 3 in 1000 live births are infected in England and Wales each year. CMV is a DNA virus of the herpes group and it is spread venereally by the oropharyngeal route, or by blood transfusion.

Maternal illness

Usually symptomless, therefore diagnosis is retrospective following discovery of a congenitally infected infant. Fifty per cent of adults have antibodies to CMV. Fetal infection may follow primary maternal infection or reactivation of maternal infection.

Fetal effects

Diagnosis is made by isolation of the virus from urine or a throat swab in the first few weeks of life.

Defects may follow infection at any gestation and 10% of infected infants have significant handicaps. Sensorineural deafness is the most common sequel. Acute neonatal illness (cytomegalic inclusion disease) occurs in 5% of infected infants and is associated with a high mortality.

Screening

This is not useful because congenital infection may follow reactivation of an old infection and defects may follow exposure at any gestation. Most cases of maternal CMV infection are asymptomatic.

Immunization

Immunization is not available.

TOXOPLASMOSIS

This is an infection with the protozoon *Toxoplasma gondii*. Oocysts from this organism are found in raw meat and cat faeces. This is a rare congenital infection in the UK and approximately 1 in 100 000 live births are infected.

Maternal illness

Infection is usually subclinical and only 10% of affected women have fever and lymphadenopathy.

Fetal infection is seen only after primary infection in the mother.

Fetal effects

Congenital infection occurs in 30% of infants whose mothers seroconvert during pregnancy. Stillbirth, neonatal death or severe handicap occur in 15% of these infants and late effects may occur.

Screening

Screening is not done routinely at present in the UK because toxoplasmosis is rare and diagnosis and treatment is difficult.

Treatment

Spiramycin is the drug of choice for treatment of the mother with primary infection. This may reduce the fetal infection rate.

HERPES SIMPLEX

Herpes simplex virus (HSV) is a DNA virus and is widespread in human populations. Most perinatal infections are caused by HSV type 2. Transplacental infection is rare and infection usually occurs during delivery.

Maternal illness

Genital ulceration follows primary infection by HSV type 2. Reactivation of infection may occur during pregnancy but rarely causes neonatal disease.

Fetal effects

There is a small risk of infection during delivery but the mortality from disseminated neurological disease is high.

Screening

Taking cervical swabs for the detection of HSV in later pregnancy is common practice, but their value is controversial. It is estimated that this method detects only 25% of women shedding virus at the time of delivery.

Management

This is controversial. In most centres, women with active genital lesions or positive viral cultures in later pregnancy are delivered by elective caesarean section. If membranes have been ruptured for four hours or more, the risk of infection is thought to be no greater from vaginal delivery than from caesarean section. The mortality from neonatal herpes infection has been reduced by the use of antiviral agents.

VARICELLA

Varicella (primary herpes zoster, chickenpox) is rare during pregnancy as most adults were infected during childhood.

Maternal illness

Varicella is a febrile illness with a characteristic rash and reactivation of the virus may cause shingles.

Fetal effects

Congenital varicella syndrome with characteristic skin scarring is extremely rare.

Varicella carries a high morbidity and mortality in infants who develop a rash 5–10 days after birth. However, if the rash appears before this, the illness is benign; this is because when maternal illness occurs > 7 days before delivery, maternal antibodies cross the placenta and confer passive immunity. If infection occurs after this, antibody levels are too low to be protective.

Treatment

In cases of maternal varicella at around the time of delivery, the neonate is given antivaricella zoster immune globulin.

LISTERIA

Listeriosis is caused by *Listeria monocytogenes*. This is a gram-positive bacillus which is widely distributed in the environment. It has been found in soft cheeses and prepacked foods. Listeriosis occurs in 1 in 7000 pregnancies.

Maternal effects

Non-specific febrile illness.

Fetal effects

Listeriosis is associated with spontaneous abortion, stillbirth and neonatal death.

Treatment

Ampicillin.

See also Chapter 36, Sexually transmitted diseases in pregnancy.

22. Major complications of pregnancy

PART 1
PRETERM LABOUR
A. Rodin

Expectations of the examiners

A clear understanding of this subject is essential and the candidate is expected to be able to discuss the areas of controversy in the management of this problem.

Definitions

Prematurity is defined as delivery prior to 37 completed weeks of pregnancy (WHO definition). In practical terms, most complications occur at gestations less than 34 weeks and most obstetricians would allow delivery beyond this gestation. Low birth weight infants weigh less than 2500 g at delivery and they may be preterm, growth retarded or both. Very low birth weight infants weigh less than 1500 g at delivery.

Interesting facts

Preterm labour complicates 5–10% of pregnancies and it is the major factor contributing to perinatal mortality and morbidity. Preterm delivery is responsible for 75% of all perinatal deaths and 85% of neonatal deaths not due to congenital abnormality. The diagnosis of preterm labour is difficult and up to 50% of women who complain of painful uterine contractions do not proceed to delivery.

The survival rate of preterm infants has increased in recent years and this is mainly due to advances in neonatal care. After 32 weeks, survival is almost equivalent to those infants born at term, and in most centres, survival of infants weighing > 1000 g is 70%. Preterm delivery may be associated with long-term handicap.

Pathophysiology

The mechanism of normal and preterm labour remains unknown and therefore the pathophysiology of this process remains uncertain. In about 60% of cases a cause can be identified but the remainder are idiopathic.

Causes of preterm labour

1. Maternal
   a. Pre-eclampsia
   b. Antepartum haemorrhage
   c. Chorioamnionitis
   d. Other infections, e.g. pyelonephritis
   e. Uterine abnormalities, e.g. congenital septae, cervical incompetence
   f. Polyhydramnios.
2. Fetal
   a. Multiple pregnancy
   b. Intrauterine death
   c. Congenital abnormality
   d. Growth retardation.

In addition, a number of risk factors have been identified which are thought to increase the chances of preterm labour and delivery in an individual.

Risk factors for preterm labour

1. General
   a. Low socioeconomic class
   b. Multiparity
   c. Maternal age < 20 years
   d. Low prepregnancy weight
   e. Smoking.
2. Past obstetric factors
   a. Previous preterm labour
   b. Previous low birth weight infant
   c. Previous antepartum haemorrhage.
3. Current pregnancy
   a. Threatened abortion
   b. Unexplained elevated AFP
   c. Antepartum haemorrhage.

Attempts to devise scoring systems to predict the risk of preterm delivery have been unsuccessful and the best predictor of preterm delivery is a previous preterm delivery.

Assessment

It is essential to make an accurate diagnosis of preterm labour before any intervention is initiated. A history is taken and questions are directed at finding a cause for preterm labour. Gestational age is checked. General examination is performed and the state of the cervix is assessed noting whether membranes are ruptured or intact.

Cardiotocography is used to assess fetal condition and to confirm regular uterine activity. Ultrasound examination can be used to confirm fetal presentation, to exclude major fetal abnormalities and to obtain an estimate of fetal weight.

The presence or absence of fetal breathing movements (FBM) has been suggested as an indicator of the outcome of preterm labour. It has been shown that in patients in preterm labour who show no FBMs over a 45-minute period, delivery in the next 48 hours is almost inevitable. The presence of FBMs indicates that the pregnancy is likely to continue.

The decision to attempt to stop preterm labour depends on a number of factors:

1. Gestational age
2. Cause of preterm labour
3. State of cervix and membranes
4. Maternal condition
5. Fetal condition
6. Local paediatric facilities.

Management

The use of tocolytics

Tocolytics act by inhibiting smooth muscle contractility. The most commonly used agents are the beta sympathomimetics (salbutamol, ritodrine, etc) which have the effect of reducing the concentration of free calcium ions within the myometrial cells and preventing contraction. These drugs have important maternal side-effects, including tachycardia and impaired glucose tolerance, and their use should be avoided in women with cardiac disease and insulin-dependent diabetes mellitus. Acute pulmonary oedema is a rare complication and is usually associated with fluid overload.

Other agents which have been used include alcohol, prostaglandin synthetase inhibitors, and calcium antagonists. Tocolytics have been shown to prolong pregnancy, however they have not yet been shown to improve perinatal mortality. They may be used in the short term to permit prenatal transfer or in the longer term to allow steroid-induced maturation of the fetal lungs. There is no evidence to support the use of oral sympathomimetics as prophylaxis for preterm labour.

The use of glucocorticoids

Antepartum administration of glucocorticoids reduces the incidence of respiratory distress syndrome (RDS) and mortality from RDS in infants between 28 to 32 weeks' gestation. For optimum effect, delivery should take place more than 24 hours and less than seven days after the start of treatment. A suitable regime is betamethasone 12 mg—two doses are given intramuscularly 12 hours apart. The use of steroids in the presence of ruptured membranes is controversial because of the theoretically increased risk of intrauterine infection.

Delivery

If local neonatal intensive care facilities are inadequate, consider transfer of the patient. In utero transfer is preferred to neonatal transfer.

The mode of delivery of premature infants is controversial. Generally, infants presenting by the vertex are delivered vaginally. The routine use of forceps in these cases confers no benefit and may contribute to morbidity. Elective episiotomy is generally used. There is no consensus about the safest route of delivery for preterm infants presenting by the breech.

PRETERM PREMATURE RUPTURE OF MEMBRANES (PPROM)

Definition

Rupture of the membranes before the onset of labour and before completion of the 37th week of pregnancy.

Interesting facts

PPROM occurs in up to 40% of all preterm labours.

Assessment

On admission, a history is taken and a sterile speculum examination is performed to confirm the presence of ruptured membranes. An endo-cervical swab is taken for microbiological examination.

Management

The risks of maternal and fetal infection must be balanced against the risks of prematurity and in the presence of group B streptococci or active genital herpes, delivery must be expedited regardless of gestation.

If gestation is 34 weeks or more, there is little to be gained by delay and labour should be induced if spontaneous contractions do not commence within a reasonable period of time. At earlier gestations, management is conservative and both mother and fetus are carefully monitored for signs of intrauterine infection:

1. Maternal pyrexia > 37.2°C
2. Maternal leucocytosis
3. Uterine tenderness
4. Offensive liquor
5. Fetal tachycardia
6. Raised C reactive protein.

If contractions occur, intrauterine infection must be excluded before tocolytics and steroids are administered.

SUMMARY

Preterm delivery is a major cause of perinatal morbidity and mortality. In about 40% of cases, the cause is unknown. The use of risk factors to identify at-risk pregnancies is generally unsuccessful. The risks to the mother and fetus through continuing the pregnancy must be balanced against the risks to the fetus of preterm delivery.

22 % LBW
15 % of prep
25 % AN adm
50 % after 20/40.

PART 2
HYPERTENSIVE DISORDERS
J. Rymer

Expectations of the examiners

As pre-eclampsia is one of the commonest complications of pregnancy, the examiners will expect a thorough knowledge of all aspects of the subject. They will expect you to know how to classify 'hypertension' in pregnancy.

Definition

Hypertension may be defined as:

1. Mild—two diastolic blood pressure (DBP) recordings of 90 mmHg or more four hours apart or a diastolic blood pressure 110 mmHg or more on one occasion.
2. Severe—two DBP recordings of 110 mmHg or more four hours apart, or DBP 120 mmHg or more on one occasion.

Classification (WHO, RCOG)

Gestational hypertension. Hypertension after 20 weeks, during labour or the puerperium.

Pre-eclampsia. Proteinuric ($> 0.3\,g/24$ hours) hypertension after 20 weeks' gestation.

Chronic hypertension. Hypertension before 20 weeks/pre-existing.

Chronic renal disease. Proteinuric hypertension before 20 weeks.

Unclassified. No recording before 20 weeks.

PRE-ECLAMPSIA

Definition

A pregnancy specific syndrome that is characterized by raised blood pressure with proteinuria that develops after 20 weeks' gestation and may terminate in eclampsia.

Interesting facts

Pre-eclampsia is the most important cause of IUGR in singletons with no malformations.

Cerebral haemorrhage is the major cause of maternal death in pre-eclampsia.

Pathophysiology

The aetiology is unknown, but there is thought to be an abnormality of the trophoblast or of the maternal response to the trophoblast. In normal pregnancy, sensitivity to angiotensin is lost, but in pre-eclampsia this does not occur.

High blood pressure is caused by vasoconstriction associated with decreased circulating plasma volume. The fundamental pathophysiological process affects all maternal organs with specific effects on placenta, cardiovascular, renal, clotting and nervous systems and the liver.

Assessment

Symptoms are usually absent in pre-eclampsia. However, if it is severe, the patient may complain of headache, blurred vision and epigastric pain.

On examination the woman may have high blood pressure, vasoconstriction, hyperreflexia, vomiting, oliguria, spontaneous bleeding, bruising, and signs of raised intracranial pressure. (Oedema is a normal phenomenon of pregnancy but may be gross in pre-eclampsia.)

Investigations

FBC and platelets. As mentioned above, pre-eclamptic women have a reduced plasma volume so the haemoglobin concentration will be elevated, as will the packed cell volume. With severe disease, platelet consumption occurs, and the platelet level drops. Disseminated coagulation can develop so clotting tests must be carried out.

Urea, creatinine, urate. When the renal system becomes involved there is reduced uric acid clearance, thus elevating the plasma uric acid. With worsening disease the urea and creatinine levels will also rise and renal failure may develop in severe cases.

Urine. Screening relies on dipsticks but may give false positive results if the urine is alkaline, and false negatives if the urine is highly dilute or contains proteins other than albumin. Any positive result (+1 or more) necessitates an MSU to exclude infection. The amount of proteinuria should be determined in a 24-hour collection.

Liver function tests. In the presence of proteinuria or a reduced platelet count, liver enzymes should be measured (e.g. plasma aspartate transaminase).

Ultrasound scan. As the uteroplacental circulation is impaired the fetus is at risk. Perinatal mortality increases once proteinuria is established. IUGR is more common with early onset disease.

Management

Mild disease

Admit for 48 hours for assessment.

1. Monitor mother
   a. 4-hourly BP
   b. Full blood count and platelets, and clotting function
   c. 24-hour urine for 24-hour protein estimation
   d. Serum urate
   e. Liver function tests.
2. Monitor fetus
   a. Movement chart
   b. Ultrasound scan.

If the blood pressure settles, cases of mild disease can be managed as an outpatient with daily midwife visits to check the blood pressure, and the urine for protein.

Moderate disease

As for mild disease, but inpatient rather than outpatient care is advised.

The place for drug treatment in pre-eclampsia is to gain control of the blood pressure to protect the cerebral vessels. It is a temporary inpatient measure as delivery is the definitive treatment. If antihypertensive medication is commenced it must be remembered that one of the major signs of worsening disease is masked.

Severe disease

Admit and deliver.

Do baseline investigations as above including clotting studies.

Commence antihypertensives. It is difficult to know which patients should be commenced on anticonvulsants. Hyperreflexia can be used as an indicator but is unreliable. Clonus indicates that eclampsia is imminent especially if there are more than two beats. Assess general well being, as a woman who feels well is unlikely to have an eclamptic fit.

The mode of delivery depends on the gestation, the presentation of the fetus, and the state of the cervix.

After delivery the patient is still at risk of an eclamptic fit for at least 48 hours. The clotting factors and the urine output must be watched carefully. Fluid management is difficult as the patient may be oliguric and haemo-concentrated, so a central venous pressure line is advisable.

If a clotting disorder has developed, and the platelet count is $< 100 \times 10^9/l$ an epidural is contraindicated.

Antihypertensives

Labetalol. Labetalol is an alpha and beta adrenergic blocker that causes vasodilation, bradycardia, and reduces myometrial activity. Commence with 100 mg b.d. and increase up to 2.6 g daily.

Methyldopa. Methyldopa acts centrally, decreasing the sympathetic outflow from the brain. An initial dose of 500 mg is given and then 250 mg 6-hourly to a maximum of 750 mg 6-hourly.

Hydralazine. Hydralazine is a nonspecific vasodilator that causes a reflex tachycardia, and sometimes headache. Useful for the acute reduction of blood pressure, where it can be given intravenously, e.g. 5 mg boluses given every five minutes titrated against the blood pressure (maximum of 20 mg).

Nifedipine. Nifedipine is a calcium channel blocker and vasodilator. It is useful for treating the acute rises in blood pressure. It is taken sub-lingually (10 mg) and may cause headache.

Anticonvulsants

It is difficult to identify the patients who need anticonvulsants. If there are symptoms of signs of imminent eclampsia then anticonvulsants are advisable. The purpose of anticonvulsants is to prevent fitting rather than to sedate the patient.

Phenytoin can be given orally or intravenously with an initial dose of 13 mg/kg followed by 100 mg 6-hourly. If given intravenously then a cardiac monitor should be used. Heminevrin and magnesium sulphate are relatively safe alternatives.

ECLAMPSIA

This is a serious complication of pre-elcampsia because it is associated with increased maternal and fetal morbidity and mortality.

Aetiology

Fitting is a result of brain hypoxia due to ischaemia secondary to oedema and intense vasospasm.

Management

Prevention is important and most women with severe pre-eclampsia should be commenced on anticonvulsant therapy. If fits occur, basic measures are needed to establish an airway, maintain breathing and circulation. The fit should be stopped with intravenous diazepam, the blood pressure controlled, and anticonvulsants commenced. If the fetus is still in utero delivery must be expedited. Maternal sedation is needed postpartum and should be continued for at least 48 hours. Urine output, clotting and liver function tests should be closely monitored.

ESSENTIAL HYPERTENSION

In essential hypertension, the prepregnancy blood pressure is elevated and there is an absent mid-trimester drop. Essential hypertension is one of the major predisposing factors to pre-eclampsia (5 × the risk). The majority of hypertensive women who do not develop pre-eclampsia can expect a normal perinatal outcome. The control of moderate chronic hypertension in early pregnancy does not lessen the eventual incidence of superimposed pre-eclampsia.

The general aims of antenatal care are to keep the blood pressure at a safe level, and to monitor maternal renal function. Growth of the fetus should be assessed regularly by serial ultrasound.

PART 3
RHESUS ISOIMMUNIZATION
A. Rodin

Expectations of the examiners

The candidate should have a knowledge of the pathophysiology of this uncommon complication, and the importance of anti-D prophylaxis should be understood.

Interesting facts

The incidence of rhesus isoimmunization has fallen dramatically since the introduction of anti-D prophylaxis in the late 1960s and rhesus disease is no longer a major cause of perinatal mortality and morbidity. The few cases that occur are mainly due to a failure of prophylaxis or to haemolytic disease occurring in the rhesus-positive mother with other maternal alloantibodies.

Pathophysiology

The rhesus gene is made up of three parts which may be C or c, D or d and E or e, respectively. Rhesus-negative women comprise 15% of the population and they are homozygous for d. Maternal anti-D antibodies (IgG) may form when rhesus-positive fetal cells enter the circulation of a rhesus-negative mother. This commonly occurs at delivery, but feto-maternal haemorrhage may follow other complications and procedures.

Causes of fetomaternal haemorrhage

1. Spontaneous abortion
2. Termination of pregnancy
3. Ectopic pregnancy
4. Antepartum haemorrhage
5. External cephalic version
6. Amniocentesis/chorionic villus sampling
7. Delivery
8. Manual removal of placenta.

As immunization usually occurs at the end of the woman's first pregnancy, it is the second and subsequent pregnancies which are affected by haemolytic disease. If the fetus is rhesus-positive in the next pregnancy there is a rise in maternal anti-D IgG which crosses the placenta and causes haemolysis of fetal red cells. This results in anaemia and in severe cases, hydrops fetalis.

Destruction of fetal red cells leads to a rise in unconjugated bilirubin which crosses the placenta to reach the maternal circulation and liver. Some of the unconjugated bilirubin enters the amniotic fluid where levels can be measured. After delivery, haemolysis continues and levels of unconjugated bilirubin continue to rise with a risk of kernicterus (free unconjugated bilirubin is toxic to cells of the CNS and this may be a fatal condition; surviving infants may have cerebral palsy, mental retardation and deafness).

Assessment

Assessment of the sensitized woman is aimed at determining whether treatment is necessary and when treatment should be initiated.

Past obstetric history. Severity of disease increases in successive pregnancies and this helps to plan management of the current pregnancy.

Serology. If antibodies are detected, the partner's genotype is checked and if he is rhesus-negative further action may be unnecessary if paternity is certain. If the antibody titre exceeds 4 units/ml, amniocentesis is indicated.

Amniocentesis. Amniotic fluid bilirubin concentrations correlate with the severity of haemolysis. Spectrophotometry at an optical density of 450 nm produces a peak which is directly proportional to the amount of bilirubin in the liquor. Timing depends on past history and maternal antibody levels. Action-line analysis charts are used to interpret the result and plan future management.

Fetal blood sampling. Cordocentesis provides a means of directly assessing the haematological state of the fetus.

Management

At booking, screening for irregular antibodies is performed on all women. An ultrasound scan to confirm gestation is particularly important. Early referral to a regional unit is indicated for women who have had previous affected pregnancies.

In non-sensitized rhesus-negative women, screening is repeated at 28, 32 and 36 weeks. If antibodies are detected and the partner's genotype is rhesus-positive the woman is referred to a regional unit for care. Maternal antibody levels are monitored. Further management is guided by the results of amniocentesis and/or fetal blood sampling. Premature delivery may be necessary.

Treatment

1. Plasmapheresis. This has been used to reduce the maternal circulating antibody level before intraperitoneal transfusion can be performed (< 20 weeks). This technique continues to be controversial.

2. Intrauterine transfusion
   a. Intraperitoneal
   b. Intravascular.

Blood tests at delivery

1. Maternal—Kleihauer test (see below)
2. Fetal—haemoglobin, blood grouping, Coombs test, bilirubin.

Prevention of rhesus isoimmunization

The administration of anti-D IgG to the mother within 72 hours of a fetomaternal haemorrhage will prevent isoimmunization provided it is given in sufficient quantity. The size of fetomaternal transfusion can be assessed by performing a Kleihauer test. A film of maternal blood is treated with acid and maternal cells become ghosted because of the denaturation of haemoglobin; fetal haemoglobin is resistant and so fetal and maternal red cells may be distinguished. The finding of five fetal cells per 50 high power fields corresponds with a fetomaternal transfusion of 2.5 ml. 500 i.u. of anti-D IgG will neutralize 4–5 ml of fetal blood. This dose is given to all unsensitized rhesus-negative mothers delivering at > 20 weeks' gestation. In pregnancies which terminate before this gestation 250 i.u. are sufficient.

Failure of prophylaxis may be due to failure to give any or sufficient anti-D. It may also follow silent immunization during the antenatal period. Antenatal administration of anti-D has been suggested to counter this.

SUMMARY

Rhesus isoimmunization is now an uncommon complication following the introduction of prophylactic anti-D IgG. Affected pregnancies should be supervised at regional centres.

PART 4
INTRAUTERINE GROWTH RETARDATION
A. Rodin

Expectations of the examiners

An understanding of the two patterns of growth retardation is needed. The candidate will be expected to know how this condition may be detected clinically and how the diagnosis is confirmed.

Definition

Intrauterine growth retardation (IUGR) is defined as fetal weight less than the tenth percentile for gestational age.

Interesting facts

Before the introduction of ultrasonography, IUGR could only be diagnosed at birth when the infant was found to be small for gestational age, although it may have been suspected antenatally on clinical grounds. The diagnosis of IUGR relies on accurate dating and this has been facilitated by the use of ultrasound in early pregnancy. Ethnic variations in birth-weight must be considered. Growth retarded infants have a higher perinatal mortality rate, a higher incidence of neonatal morbidity and long-term cognitive performance may be impaired when compared to normal sized infants.

Pathophysiology

The pathophysiology of IUGR differs according to its aetiology but there are two main mechanisms: 1. asymetrical growth retardation: the supply of nutrients to the fetus is inadequate to support growth and this usually results from 'placental insufficiency'. This type of IUGR usually presents in later pregnancy when fetal needs are increasing. The vital organs are protected and there is sparing of head growth initially; 2. symmetrical growth retardation: this occurs when the growth potential of the fetus is reduced, for example, it may be due to chromosomal abnormalities or intrauterine infection. This type of IUGR usually appears early in pregnancy.

IUGR may be associated with oligohydramnios.

Aetiology

1. Maternal
   a. Pre-eclampsia/hypertension
   b. Placental abruption
   c. Diabetes mellitus
   d. Renal disease
   e. Smoking
   f. Alcohol
   g. Infections.
2. Fetal
   a. Chromosomal abnormalities
   b. Sickle cell disease
   c. Achondroplasia
   d. Potter's syndrome

  e. Anencephaly
  f. Multiple pregnancy.

IUGR may be idiopathic. It is associated with low socioeconomic class and may recur in subsequent pregnancies.

Assessment

An ultrasound scan is performed routinely at 18–20 weeks to confirm gestation. Some women will be in a high-risk group because of pre-existing medical disease or a past history of IUGR. Fetal growth in this group should be checked by serial ultrasound scans. In others, detection of IUGR depends on a high index of clinical suspicion. Maternal weight gain is a poor indicator of fetal growth.

On examination the uterus may be small for dates and there may be oligohydramnios. Measurement of symphysis-fundal height is a sensitive test for IUGR and when this is abnormal an ultrasound scan should be arranged.

The parameters used in ultrasound growth assessment are biparietal diameter (BPD) (Fig. 22.1), head circumference (HC), abdominal circumference (AC) (Fig. 22.2) and femur length (FL) (Fig. 22.3). In addition, liquor volume should be noted. In symmetrical IUGR, growth in all measured parameters is uniformly decreased. In asymmetrical IUGR,

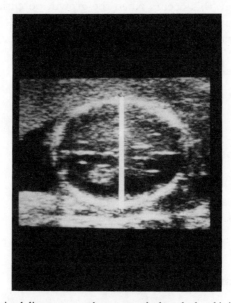

Fig. 22.1 The biparietal diameter must be measured when the head is in the occipito-transverse position, i.e. with the midline echo from the fetal brain at right angles to the ultrasound beam.

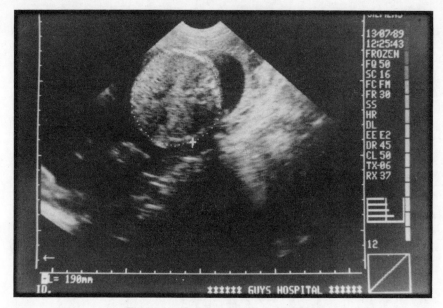

Fig. 22.2   The abdominal circumference.

rate of growth of the fetal abdomen is slowed while head growth remains normal. The role of Doppler flow studies in the assessment of the growth-retarded fetus is being evaluated.

Investigations

In symmetrical IUGR a TORCH screen should be performed and fetal karyotyping may be indicated.

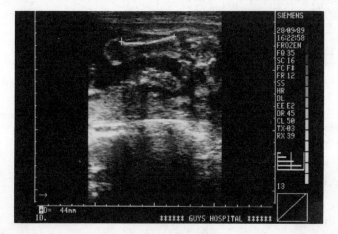

Fig. 22.3   Femur length is visualized on ultrasound scan and then measured.

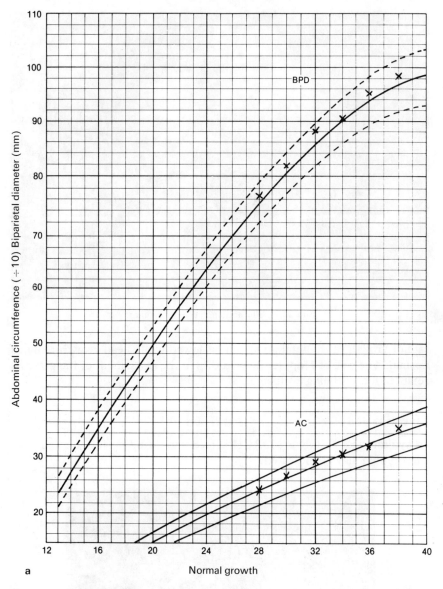

Fig. 22.4 Ultrasound measurements plotted on fetal growth charts. **a.** Normal growth; **b.** asymmetrical IUGR.

Management

Once the diagnosis of IUGR has been made, hospital admission is arranged so that the condition of both mother and fetus can be monitored. History should be reviewed and a physical examination should be performed.

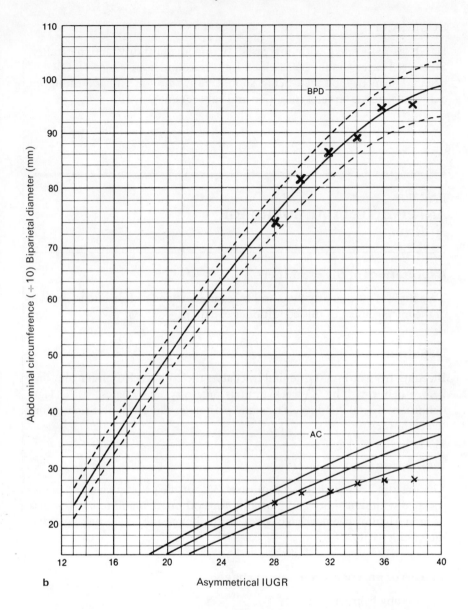

b   Asymmetrical IUGR

Growth scans are repeated every two weeks. Fetal well-being is assessed by monitoring of fetal movements and cardiotocography. Biochemical tests of placental function are no longer used routinely. In the future, Doppler flow studies and blood gas analysis of fetal blood obtained by cordocentesis may contribute to the management of these cases. Timing of delivery is usually determined by fetal well-being. In some cases, delivery is prompted by a deterioration in maternal condition.

SUMMARY

IUGR is associated with increased perinatal morbidity and mortality. Suspected cases should be assessed by ultrasound scan. Once IUGR has been confirmed, fetal well-being should be monitored and the timing of delivery depends on fetal condition and subsequent growth.

PART 5
ANTEPARTUM HAEMORRHAGE
A. Rodin

Expectations of the examiners

This topic is particularly favoured by examiners and a clear understanding of the management of this condition is essential.

Definition

Bleeding from or into the genital tract after the 28th week of pregnancy and before delivery. The 28-week limit is arbitrary and relates to the legal definition of fetal viability. The same pathology can cause bleeding before the 28th week.

Interesting facts

Antepartum haemorrhage complicates 3% of all pregnancies and is associated with morbidity and mortality for both mother and fetus. The risk of antepartum haemorrhage rises with increasing maternal age and increasing parity.

Causes of antepartum haemorrhage

1. Bleeding from the placenta
   a. Placental abruption
   b. Placenta praevia
   c. Bleeding from placental margin.
2. Bleeding from other sites
   a. Local causes, e.g. cervical polyp, cervical ectropion, cervical carcinoma
   b. Vasa praevia (rare)
   c. Unknown.

PLACENTAL ABRUPTION

Bleeding occurs due to separation of the placenta before delivery of the infant. This can vary in severity from a minor separation to complete placental detachment. The amount of vaginal bleeding does not correlate with the degree of placental separation and there may be total separation with no revealed bleeding.

Pathophysiology

Rupture of one or more maternal spiral arterioles occurs in the decidua basalis. The bleeding may be limited with the formation of a decidual haematoma. If bleeding continues, any or all of the following may occur: 1. blood may track under the placenta extending the degree of placental separation and compromising the fetus; 2. blood may dissect under the membranes to reach the cervix and vagina; and 3. blood may enter the amniotic cavity or infiltrate between the fibres of the myometrium triggering an intense inflammatory response and discolouring the uterus (couvelaire uterus). Minor separation of the placental edge may ocurr but presentation is less dramatic than frank abruption.

Following major placental abruption there is release of thromboplastin into the maternal circulation which may trigger disseminated intravascular coagulation (DIC). Maternal death following abruption is usually associated with DIC.

Aetiology

The aetiology of placental abruption is unknown. It may occur following trauma or after sudden uterine decompression which may occur when membranes rupture in a case of polyhydramnios. Abruption is associated with low socioeconomic class, hypertension, pre-eclampsia and previous abruption. The risk of placental abruption is increased in women who smoke during pregnancy.

Assessment

The clinical picture is determined by the extent of the abruption. Continuous abdominal pain is the most constant feature and is usually of sudden onset. Abruption may precipitate labour. Vaginal bleeding may occur. The patient may be shocked and the uterus is tender and tense on palpation. It may be difficult to feel fetal parts and the fetal heart sounds may be absent. The differential diagnosis includes other causes of pain and bleeding in pregnancy.

Placental abruption is diagnosed clinically. Investigations are aimed at monitoring fetal and maternal well-being.

Management (see also General management of antepartum haemorrhage)

When a firm diagnosis of abruption is made delivery is indicated. The diagnosis is sometimes difficult, particularly prior to 34 weeks gestation. If the woman is in labour and there is no evidence of fetal or maternal compromise then the membranes should be ruptured, otherwise caesarean section is usually indicated.

PLACENTA PRAEVIA

The placenta is low-lying in 20% of pregnancies at the end of the second trimester but the incidence falls with advancing gestation as the lower segment forms. Placenta pravia complicates approximately 0.5% of pregnancies at term, however a significant proportion deliver before this. Abruption may occur in placenta praevia.

Aetiology

The aetiology of placenta praevia is unknown but previous myometrial damage (e.g. following curettage) has been implicated. Placenta praevia is commoner in pregnancies after caesarean section and if it occurs the possibility of pathological adherence of the placenta must be anticipated. There is an association with multiple pregnancy and rhesus disease where the placental area is larger.

Assessment

Painless recurrent vaginal bleeding is the characteristic symptom of placenta praevia, however in some cases bleeding does not occur until the onset of labour. On examination, the uterus is not tender and there may be a breech presentation, abnormal lie or the presenting part may be high. These findings should raise the suspicion of placenta praevia even in the absence of vaginal bleeding. *Vaginal examination must not be performed if placenta praevia is suspected.*

Investigations

Placental localization is performed by ultrasound. This technique is usually accurate but is not infallible. There are four grades of placenta praevia:

Grade 1: Lower margin of placenta encroaches on the lower segment
Grade 2: Lower margin of placenta reaches the internal os
Grade 3: Placenta partially covers the internal os
Grade 4: Placenta completely covers the internal os.

Placenta praevia is more simply classified into major and minor degrees.

A minor degree of placenta praevia is equivalent to grade 1 or 2, and a major degree corresponds with grades 3 and 4.

Management

If a low-lying placenta is detected by routine scan in early pregnancy no action is necessary, but the placental site is checked again at 32 weeks' gestation. If a major degree of placenta praevia persists the patient is admitted to hospital because of the risk of haemorrhage. Crossmatched blood is kept continuously available and ultrasound scans are repeated at 2-week intervals to monitor placental position and fetal growth.

If a major degree of placenta praevia persists at 38 weeks, delivery is by elective caesarean section. This should be performed by a senior obstetrician and general anaesthesia is advised. Women with minor degrees of placenta praevia would usually be allowed to labour spontaneously. Examination under anaesthesia is rarely indicated.

Other causes of antepartum haemorrhage

Vasa praevia is a rare condition and can occur when there is a velamentous cord insertion. The cord inserts in the membranes and the vessels course across the membranes to reach the placenta. When membranes rupture the vessels may be torn and fetal exsanguination may occur. Facilities should be available to test for fetal haemoglobin.

General management of antepartum haemorrhage

Management depends primarily on the severity of the clinical situation. It is obligatory to assume that bleeding is placental in origin until proven otherwise.

Minor haemorrhage

At home

1. Refer patient to hospital
2. *Do not perform a vaginal examination.*

In hospital

1. Take a history and examine the patient
2. *Do not perform a digital vaginal examination*
3. Gentle speculum examination may be performed after the placental site is known
4. Assess fetal well-being—cardiotocography
5. Consider siting an intravenous line

6. Take blood to check haemoglobin, platelets and group and save serum
7. Admit to hospital for rest and observation
8. Arrange ultrasound scan
9. Give anti-D to rhesus-negative mothers.

Major haemorrhage

At home

1. Arrange urgent admission to hospital/call obstetric flying squad
2. Insert intravenous line and commence resuscitation
3. *Do not perform a vaginal examination.*

In hospital

1. Call for assistance
2. Insert wide-bore cannula and commence intravenous infusion; two lines may be necessary
3. Request six units of crossmatched blood urgently
4. Send blood to check haemoglobin, platelets and clotting screen
5. Insert CVP line
6. Insert urinary catheter; monitor fluid balance
7. *Do not perform a vaginal examination*
8. If the fetus is alive, deliver by emergency caesarean section.

Complications of antepartum haemorrhage

1. Maternal/fetal death
2. Postpartum haemorrhage
3. DIC (particularly following abruption)
4. Renal failure
5. Preterm delivery.

SUMMARY

Placental abruption and placenta praevia are the important causes of antepartum haemorrhage. Assessment in hospital is essential in all cases of antepartum haemorrhage and management is determined by the clinical situation.

PART 6
MATERNAL SYSTEMIC DISORDERS
A. Rodin

Expectations of the examiners

The candidate is expected to have a knowledge of the common medical disorders which occur in pregnancy. The candidate should be able to discuss the role of the general practitioner in their management.

ANAEMIA

Interesting facts

Anaemia is one of the commonest medical complications of pregnancy.

Pathophysiology

Plasma volume increases steadily through pregnancy and reaches a plateau after 32 weeks. The magnitude of the increase is related to fetal size and the effect is exaggerated in multiple pregnancy. There is a concomitant increase in red cell mass and total haemoglobin but because of the larger rise in plasma volume, the haemoglobin concentration and PCV fall.

IRON DEFICIENCY ANAEMIA

Demands for iron increase during pregnancy due to the rise in red cell mass and fetal demands. Total iron requirement through pregnancy is 700–1400 mg with a daily requirement of 4 mg rising to 7 mg in later pregnancy. A reduction in haemoglobin concentration is a relatively late sign of iron deficiency. This is preceeded by depletion in iron stores and a fall in serum iron levels.

Assessment

Iron deficiency can be detected before anaemia develops by measuring serum ferritin which gives a reflection of iron stores. Serum iron and total iron binding capacity are also useful markers.

The red cell indices suggestive of iron deficiency are reduced mean cell volume (MCV) and a reduced mean cell haemoglobin concentration (MCHC).

Management

Oral iron supplements are usually adequate for prophylaxis. Standard preparations contain between 100–200 mg of elemental iron often in combination with folic acid.

Treatment of established iron deficiency depends on the severity of the anaemia and the gestation. Treatment options include:

1. Oral iron supplementation
2. Parenteral iron/dextran (i.v./i.m.) $\left.\right\}$ Rarely needed
3. Blood transfusion.

Adequate treatment should increase the haemoglobin concentration at the rate of 1 mg/dl/week and a reticulocyte count 2 weeks later should confirm a response to iron therapy.

MEGALOBLASTIC ANAEMIA

A deficiency in folic acid is the usual cause of this type of anaemia in pregnancy. Folate is needed for cell growth and division and requirements increase as pregnancy progresses. Folate deficiency anaemia affects 5% of pregnant women in the UK and much larger numbers in developing countries. The daily requirement of folate in pregnancy is 100 μg.

Assessment

The red cell indices show a raised MCV and macrocytes are seen on the blood film.

Management

Oral folate supplements, 5 mg daily for documented folate deficiency, are often combined with iron supplements. Prophylactic dose is 200–500 μg of folate.

SICKLE CELL ANAEMIA

Sickle cell disease is one of the most important haemoglobinopathies. It is due to a single amino acid substitution on the beta chain of haemoglobin. The haemoglobin formed (HbS) is insoluble when reduced and this results in distortion of erythrocytes and subsequent blockage of small blood vessels. Sickle cell disease is common amongst black populations and in some Mediterranean groups. Heterozygotes for this abnormal gene have sickle cell trait (HbAS). Complications in pregnancy are rare. Homozygotes (HbSS) have sickle cell disease and may suffer from recurrent sickling crises. They develop a chronic haemolytic anaemia.

Assessment

Sickle cell disease and other haemoglobinopathies are detected by haemo-globin electrophoresis which should be carried out in at-risk women at booking. The partner's blood should also be tested to assess the risks of fetal disease.

Management

Women with sickle cell trait pose few special management problems. Haemoglobin electrophoresis should be performed on the baby's father to assess risks of the infant being affected.

Women with sickle cell disease should be managed in specialist centres and further discussion is beyond the scope of this book.

CARDIAC DISEASE

Interesting facts

Less than 1% of all pregnancies in the UK are complicated by heart disease, however it remains an important cause of maternal mortality. Greater numbers of women with congenital heart disease are now reaching adulthood due to paediatric cardiac surgery and many of these women are becoming pregnant. The numbers of women with acquired (mainly rheumatic) heart disease complicating pregnancy are falling.

Pathophysiology

During normal pregnancy the cardiovascular system undergoes a number of adaptations. During the first trimester cardiac output increases by 40% due to raised stroke volume and a small increment in heart rate. Blood volume also increases by about 40% in early pregnancy and this is maintained until term. A fall in peripheral resistance occurs due to general relaxation in arterial and venous tone. An ejection systolic murmur is audible in up to 90% of normal pregnant women. At delivery, contraction of the uterus expresses about 500 ml of blood into the circulation. The normal woman can cope with these haemodynamic alterations but in a woman with heart disease they may precipitate cardiac failure.

Classification of heart disease

1. Congenital heart disease
2. Rheumatic heart disease
3. Other
   a. Cardiomyopathy
   b. Myocardial infarction.

Maternal mortality is most likely in those conditions where pulmonary blood flow cannot be increased, e.g. Eisenmenger's syndrome and primary pulmonary hypertension. Fetal outcome in patients with rheumatic heart disease and acyanotic congenital heart disease is usually good. Mothers with cyanotic congenital heart disease tend to have growth retarded infants.

Although rheumatic heart disease is becoming rare in the UK it is the commonest form of heart disease complicating pregnancy worldwide. The most important lesion is mitral stenosis and these women are particularly likely to develop heart failure during pregnancy.

Women with artificial heart valves should receive anticoagulation through pregnancy and the puerperium.

Management

Prepregnancy

Avoidance or termination of pregnancy may be recommended in certain conditions (e.g. Eisenmenger's syndrome).

Antenatal

1. Hospital care with regular visits to obstetrician and cardiologist
2. Avoid cardiac failure
   a. Treat infections promptly
   b. Treat hypertension
   c. Avoid anaemia
3. Treat cardiac failure
4. Monitor fetal growth with serial ultrasound scans.

In labour

1. Antibiotic cover may be indicated
2. Aim for vaginal delivery
3. Adequate analgesia—epidural analgesia can be used in most cases but should be avoided in women with Eisenmenger's syndrome and hypertrophic cardiomyopathy (i.e. fixed output states)
4. Strict control of intravenous fluids
5. Short second stage
6. Do not give ergometrine.

DIABETES MELLITUS

Interesting facts

Diabetes affects about 3% of the obstetric population and before the introduction of insulin, diabetic pregnancy had a very high maternal and fetal mortality.

Pathophysiology

Hormonal changes during pregnancy have profound effects on carbohydrate metabolism. Insulin resistance develops as pregnancy advances and it is most marked in the last trimester. In normal pregnancy, increased insulin production counters the rise in insulin resistance and blood glucose levels are maintained within a narrow range. Glucose crosses the placenta freely by facilitated diffusion and maternal homeostatic mechanisms regulate fetal glucose levels in the normal situation. In the diabetic pregnancy, fetal hyperglycaemia stimulates fetal insulin production.

Glycosuria is common during normal pregnancy. This is due to an increased glomerular filtration rate and reduced tubular reabsorption of glucose.

There are three main clinical types of diabetes in pregnancy:

1. Insulin-dependent diabetes
2. Non-insulin dependent diabetes
3. Gestational diabetes.

Gestational diabetes is the term applied to women who become diabetic during pregnancy. Many will revert to normal after pregnancy, but a proportion do not.

Effects of diabetes on the pregnancy

Fetal effects

1. Increased perinatal mortality due to:
   a. Congenital abnormalities: increased risk of sacral agenesis and cardiac abnormalities due to hyperglycaemia during organogenesis.
   b. Respiratory distress syndrome
   c. Birth trauma associated with macrosomia (birth weight > 4000 g)
   d. Intrauterine growth retardation
   e. Prematurity.
2. Increased neonatal morbidity
   a. Birth asphyxia/trauma
   b. Hypoglycaemia
   c. Polycythaemia
   d. Jaundice
   e. Respiratory distress syndrome.

Maternal effects

1. Pre-eclampsia: increased incidence in diabetic pregnancy
2. Polyhydramnios
3. Preterm labour.

Good diabetic control reduces the incidence of these complications but the raised incidence of congenital abnormalities persists.

Assessment

Risk factors should be identified antenatally and these women should be offered a glucose tolerance test.

Risk factors for gestational diabetes are:

1. Glycosuria on two or more occasions
2. Maternal obesity ($>20\%$ of ideal weight)
3. Family history of diabetes in first degree relative
4. Previous congenital abnormality, neonatal death, unexplained stillbirth, macrosomic infant
5. Polyhydramnios in current pregnancy
6. Previous gestational diabetes.

Routine antenatal screening is recommended by some because about 30% of gestational diabetics have none of these risk factors.

The diagnosis of diabetes is made by the finding of a fasting blood glucose level of 8 mmol/l or more or 11 mmol/l or more after food. A fasting glucose level of <6 mmol/l excludes the diagnosis. A glucose tolerance test (GTT) with a 75 g glucose load distinguishes between diabetes, impaired glucose tolerance (IGT) and normality. The significance of IGT to the pregnancy is uncertain but some women with IGT will develop gestational diabetes later in the pregnancy.

Management

Medical management of diabetes is by diet alone or diet and insulin depending on the type of maternal diabetes. Oral hypoglycaemic agents are not used. Insulin is given at least twice daily using a mixture of short-acting and medium-acting preparations. Continuous subcutaneous insulin administration has been used with good effect.

Prepregnancy

Established diabetics should be assessed before pregnancy to achieve optimal blood glucose control before conception. Women with diabetic retinopathy and nephropathy require careful assessment.

Antenatal

1. Early booking
2. Hospital care at joint obstetric/diabetic clinic
3. Optimize blood glucose control

    a. Dietary advice
    b. Home blood glucose monitoring
    c. Regular urinalysis
    d. Regular HbA1 and fructosamine monitoring
4. Monitor fetal well-being
    a. Check maternal serum AFP between 16–18 weeks
    b. Anomaly scan at 18 weeks
    c. Serial ultrasound scans to monitor fetal growth
5. Do not allow pregnancy to proceed past 40 weeks.

In labour

1. Aim for vaginal delivery
2. Continuous intravenous infusion of insulin and 5% dextrose with regular monitoring of blood glucose
3. Continuous fetal monitoring
4. Adequate analgesia.

After delivery, insulin requirements fall rapidly and careful monitoring is essential.

EPILEPSY

Interesting facts

Pregnancy does not trigger epilepsy or cause an exacerbation of pre-existing epilepsy. Untreated epileptics have an increased risk of congenital abnormalities which is poorly understood. The incidence of congenital malformations is increased 2- or 3-fold in infants of women on anti-convulsants. Phenytoin is associated with an increased risk of cleft lip/palate, congenital heart disease and hypoplasia of the nails and digits. Sodium valproate is associated with an increased incidence of neural tube defects.

Management

Prepregnancy

1. Check that fits are well controlled
2. Emphasize the importance of good drug compliance during pregnancy.

Antenatal

1. Continue on usual anticonvulsant at prepregnancy dose unless fits occur then levels should be checked and the dose adjusted accordingly.
2. Women taking anticonvulsants may become folate deficient and 5 mg daily should be given throughout pregnancy.

3. Maternal serum AFP estimation at 16–18 weeks.
4. Fetal anomaly scan at 18 weeks.
5. Anticonvulsants may cause depression of vitamin K-dependent clotting factors in the mother and fetus; vitamin K should be given from 36 weeks until delivery and the neonate should be given vitamin K intramuscularly.

THROMBOEMBOLIC DISEASE

Interesting facts

Thromboembolic disease is an important cause of maternal mortality. The risk of thromboembolism during pregnancy and the puerperium is six times higher than in the non-pregnant state.

Pathophysiology

Pregnancy is accompanied by changes in normal haemostatic mechanisms which decrease the risk of haemorrhage at delivery. These changes include an increase in clotting factors and a dampening of fibrinolysis favouring thrombosis. Risk factors for thromboembolism in pregnancy include:

1. High maternal age
2. Multiparity
3. Obesity
4. Immobility
5. Previous history of thromboembolism
6. Operative delivery
7. Blood disorders (rare)
8. Use of stilboestrol to suppress lactation.

Blood group O appears to confer some protection against thromboembolism. The recurrence rate of deep venous thrombosis (DVT) or pulmonary embolus (PE) in women who have had thromboembolic disease in previous pregnancies is 5–10%.

Assessment

Women with a history of thromboembolism should be identified in the booking clinic. Suspected thromboembolism occurring during pregnancy or the puerperium should be actively investigated to reach a definitive diagnosis. Clinical diagnosis of DVT is unreliable and venography or ultrasonography should be arranged. Clinical suspicion of PE should be confirmed by a ventilation-perfusion scan of the lungs. Chest X-ray, ECG and arterial blood gas measurement may also be helpful. Anticoagulation should be commenced when thromboembolism is suspected without waiting for confirmation.

Management

PE/DVT during pregnancy

1. Commence intravenous infusion of heparin 40 000 i.u./day; continue for 5–7 days.
2. Change to subcutaneous heparin 10 000 i.u. b.d. and continue until the end of the puerperium.

History of previous DVT/PE

Prophylactic anticoagulation should be considered because of risk of recurrence. There is no consensus about who to treat and which regime to follow and the benefits of anticoagulation should be balanced against the risks of fetal and maternal side-effects (see below). Regimes which have been used include:

1. Continuous subcutaneous heparin through pregnancy and the puerperium
2. Subcutaneous heparin until 13 weeks; warfarin between 13–36 weeks; subcutaneous heparin from 36 weeks until the end of the puerperium
3. Dextran 70 in labour followed by heparin (subcutaneous) or warfarin during the puerperium.

Anticoagulation with either heparin or warfarin is associated with risks for both mother and fetus. Heparin does not cross the placenta and it has a short half-life. Its actions are readily reversible by protamine sulphate. However, it is associated with maternal thrombocytopenia and prolonged administration causes bone demineralization. Warfarin crosses the placenta and can cause chondrodysplasia punctata, microcephaly and optic atrophy in the fetus. Later in pregnancy it can cause fetal intracranial haemorrhage. Therefore warfarin is avoided in the first trimester and from 36 weeks onwards. Warfarin has a long half-life and its effects cannot be rapidly reversed in the event of a complication such as antepartum haemorrhage. Breast-feeding is not contraindicated in women taking heparin or warfarin.

THYROID DISEASE

Interesting facts

Thyroid disease has been estimated to complicate 0.5% of all pregnancies. It is usually pre-existing but may appear for the first time in pregnancy.

HYPOTHYROIDISM

The main causes of hypothyroidism are idiopathic, Hashimoto's thyroiditis and postablative hypothyroidism.

Assessment

The clinical diagnosis of hypothyroidism may be difficult during pregnancy but may be suggested by inappropriate weight gain, cold intolerance or skin changes. There may be a goitre and reflexes may be sluggish. Laboratory investigations show a low free thyroxine (T4) level and a raised thyroid stimulating hormone (TSH) level. Total serum T4 is low for pregnancy but may be within the normal range for the non-pregnant woman.

Management

Thyroxine should be given as a single daily dose. Thyroid function should be checked as the pregnancy progresses. Breast-feeding is not contra-indicated.

HYPERTHYROIDISM

Hyperthyroidism in pregnancy is usually due to Grave's disease. Untreated hyperthyroidism is associated with increased incidence of preterm labour and low birth-weight and a raised perinatal mortality rate. Women who have had surgery for Grave's disease may still have thyroid stimulating autoantibodies which can cross the placenta and cause neonatal thyrotoxicosis.

Assessment

The symptoms of hyperthyroidism may mimic the normal changes of pregnancy and include heat intolerance, palpitations, emotional lability and fatigue. A goitre may be present. TSH is undetectable while free T3 and T4 are elevated.

Management

The aim of management is to control maternal hyperthyroidism while allowing the development of normal thyroid function in the fetus. Both drug therapy and surgery have been used. The thiourea derivatives, carbimazole and propylthiouracil are in common use and their main action is to inhibit synthesis of T3 and T4. These drugs cross the placenta and may effect the fetal thyroid causing transient hypothyroidism at delivery. There is no contraindication to breast-feeding.

23. Labour—first stage

J. Rymer

Expectations of the examiners

The candidate is expected to understand the mechanism of labour and the management of normal and abnormal labour. The principles of active management of labour are essential to modern obstetrics.

Definitions

Labour is defined as the process by which the fetus, placenta, and membranes are expelled from the birth canal. The first stage of labour commences when regular uterine contractions are associated with cervical change, and concludes with full dilatation of the cervix.

Interesting facts

Previously labour was said to be normal when spontaneous delivery occurred within 24 hours of the onset of spontaneous regular contractions. However, as the complications of labour are directly related to its duration, labour is now deemed normal if spontaneous delivery occurs within 12 hours.

Physiology

In pregnancy, the uterus is in a relaxed state and must expand to accommodate the growing fetus. However, when labour commences, it must contract regularly and forcibly so that the cervix progressively effaces and dilates allowing the fetus to descend through the birth canal.

In labour, the myometrial smooth muscle contracts at regular intervals, resulting in intrauterine pressures of 50–75 mmHg. The wave of excitation, and hence the resulting contraction normally passes downwards from the fundus of the uterus. As the muscle contracts, it also retracts (the muscle does not relax to its original length, but stays at a shorter length). Successful parturition involves regular and effective uterine contractions and a responsive cervix. Cervical ripening is characterized by softening, effacement and dilatation, but the hormonal control of this process is still not understood. Prior to term, the release of prostaglandins causes an increase in the water content of the cervix and breakdown of cervical collagen. PGE2 has a marked effect on cervical ripening. During labour, prostaglandins and oxytocin interact in the generation of uterine contractions.

Mechanism of normal labour

Descent. Significant descent of the head into the pelvis occurs in most primigravidae in the later weeks of pregnancy. In multigravidae descent may not occur until the onset of labour.

Engagement. This occurs when the maximum diameter of the head has passed through the pelvic brim. It may occur before labour commences, and the head usually engages in the occipito-transverse. (See Appendix.)

Flexion. This is a continuous process during labour. With full flexion the posterior fontanelle is easily palpable on vaginal examination through the dilated cervix, and the most favourable diameter presents.

Internal rotation. This is rotation of the head inside the pelvis, and it occurs because of the shape of the birth canal, the position of the head, and the inclination of the levator ani. Usually the rotation is anterior, so that the denominator (the occiput) swings from LOT to direct OA.

Extension. The head remains flexed until the vertex reaches the perineum. As the head 'crowns' it extends, following the axis of the birth canal.

External rotation (restitution). The head reverts to the position it previously held before internal rotation occurred (occipito-transverse).

Lateral flexion. The anterior shoulder appears, followed by the posterior shoulder. Delivery of the trunk is then achieved by lateral flexion.

Assessment

The diagnosis of labour is made when regular uterine contractions are associated with cervical change. As the cervix effaces the operculum (mucus plug in the cervix) is released (a 'show'). Each obstetric unit should be clear on its criteria for the diagnosis of labour, and the delivery suite should be reserved for women in active labour.

History

Specific questioning should involve:

1. Contractions
   a. Time of onset
   b. Frequency
   c. Duration

2. Presence of a show
3. Ruptured membranes.

Examination

1. Abdominal palpation is performed to assess:
   a. Gestation
   b. Lie of the fetus
   c. Presentation
   d. Descent of the head (Fig. 23.1).
2. Vaginal examination:
   a. Speculum examination if there is any question as to whether liquor is draining. Nitrazene reaction has been used to indicate the presence of liquor but is unreliable.
   b. Digital examination should assess the softness, length, and dilatation of the cervix, and the station (relative to the ischial spines) of the presenting part.
3. Fetal well-being:
   a. Fetal movements
   b. CTG (ideally for 20 minutes)
   c. Presence of meconium in the liquor.

Management

If the diagnosis of 'labour' is made then the membranes should be ruptured provided that a cord presentation has been excluded. This enables the colour of the liquor to be assessed, and aids the progress of labour. The best way to record the progress of labour is to use a partogram, i.e. a visual representation of progress in labour. This should include a record of:

1. The date and time of admission
2. Cervical dilatation. This is marked in centimetres at zero time (on admission) and at subsequent examinations
3. Descent of the head. Can be determined by vaginal assessment of the relationship of the presenting part to the ischial spines (station) and abdominal palpation of the number of 'fifths' of the head palpable above the brim
4. Contractions
   a. Frequency
   b. Duration
   c. Strength: assessment of strength of contractions by palpation is unreliable
5. Fetal heart rate
6. Colour of the liquor and time and manner of membrane rupture
7. The use of syntocinon

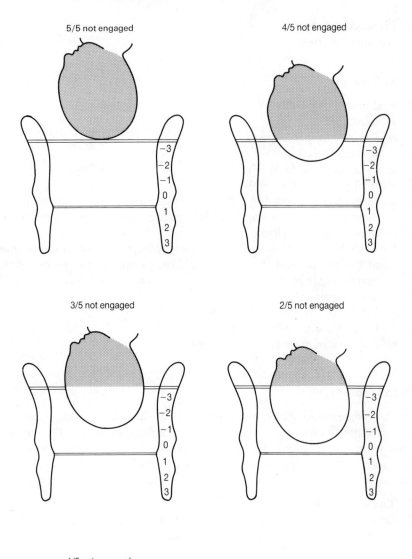

1/5 not engaged

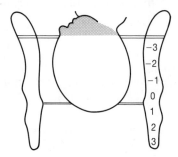

Fig. 23.1 The abdominal palpation of the fetal head can be described in 'fifths' of the head palpable above the brim.

8. Maternal status
   a. Blood pressure
   b. Pulse
   c. Temperature
   d. Urinalysis
   e. Medication.

Progress in labour

The regular assessment of progress is the key to good management. In primigravidae, delivery should be achieved within 12 hours. The minimum rate of cervical dilatation acceptable in primiparous women is 1 cm/hour. Delay in progress may be due to:

Inefficient uterine action (primary dysfunctional labour). In primiparous women this is common. The earlier the diagnosis is made the more chance there is of correcting it and achieving a normal delivery. Once diagnosed, a syntocinon infusion should be commenced and progress assessed regularly. (See Appendix VII for Partograms.)

Secondary arrest. If the fetal head is partially extended it does not fit into the lower uterine pole well and this is more common in primiparous women especially with an occipito-posterior position. These women generally have a bad start to labour, and may present with inefficient uterine action. Premature rupture of membranes is common. The head remains high and deflexed and there may be severe backache. The sinciput reaches the pelvic floor first and therefore rotates anteriorly, i.e. the occiput is posterior. The larger occipito-frontal diameter of the head presents (10 cm) making its passage through the pelvis more difficult.

Cephalopelvic disproportion. (See Ch. 24.) In multiparous women, labour is more rapid and inefficient uterine action is less common. Delay in a multiparous woman may be due to obstruction with subsequent uterine rupture if not recognized.

Posture during labour

The woman should adopt the most comfortable position bearing in mind that aorto-caval compression must be avoided.

Oral intake

Women in labour have delayed gastric emptying and this will be exacerbated by narcotics and fatigue. It is advisable to allow clear fluids and no food. H2 antagonists should be given 6 hourly.

Support during labour

Labour is a stressful event and a woman requires support from a person known to her and a midwife who ideally remains with her throughout her labour.

Active management of labour

The aim of active management is to ensure that all women in their first pregnancy deliver a healthy child after a labour less than 12 hours. A woman's first experience will determine her obstetric future both emotionally and physically.

The principles of active management are:

1. Antenatal education
2. Regular assessment of progress in labour
3. Presence of a support person throughout labour (ideally, the *same* person throughout)
4. Early correction of abnormal progress
5. Provision of suitable analgesia.

If active management is correctly applied, the caesarean section rate is reduced.

24. Labour—second stage

J. Rymer

Expectations of the examiners

The candidate will be expected to have a thorough knowledge of what is normal and abnormal in the second stage of labour. The importance of the correct timing of intervention should be appreciated.

Definition

The second stage of labour commences with full cervical dilatation and concludes with delivery of the fetus.

Interesting facts

In primigravidae the average length of the second stage is 40 minutes, and in multiparae, 20 minutes.

Physiology

The uterus continues to contract and force the fetus through the cervix. At full dilatation the cervix has retracted past the presenting part and is no longer palpable. Contractions are usually stronger but occur less frequently than in the first stage. If the normal mechanism of labour is occurring, the head rotates internally as it descends and when the pelvic floor becomes distended the 'bearing down' reflex occurs.

Assessment

Full dilatation is diagnosed by vaginal examination. The position and station of the fetal head should be noted.

Management

When the bearing down reflex occurs the woman will want to 'push' (in the absence of an effective epidural). After breathing in, the glottis is closed, and the patient pushes down with the aid of the diaphragm and abdominal wall muscles. Two or three bearing down efforts are made with each contraction. It is essential that the woman receives constant attention during the second stage to detect signs of fetal or maternal distress.

Once anal dilatation occurs, normal delivery should follow shortly afterwards. The woman is prepared for delivery, and the accoucheur assists the delivery by ensuring that the fetal head remains flexed, and that the head is delivered in a controlled manner. If needed, an episiotomy is performed (ideally with some form of pain relief) as the head distends the perineum. Once the head is delivered the oropharynx is suctioned. The head restitutes and is then grasped and pulled downwards (towards the maternal sacrum) so that the anterior shoulder is delivered. The trunk is then laterally flexed upwards (towards the maternal umbilicus) so that the posterior shoulder is delivered, rapidly followed by the trunk. Great care of the perineum must be taken at all times.

If a spontaneous vaginal delivery has not occurred within one hour of full dilatation then the vaginal examination should be repeated. In primigravida women, if there has been no progress, then a syntocinon infusion should be commenced and a repeat vaginal examination should be performed in one hour. If there is no progress and the head is too high for a forceps delivery, then a caesarean section is performed. If progress has occurred, then an instrumental delivery may be performed, or the second stage may be allowed to continue depending on the fetal and maternal condition. In multiparous women, it is dangerous to use syntocinon for second stage augmentation alone, due to the risk of uterine rupture.

If the position of the head is occipito-anterior and does not descend with augmentation (in primigravidae) this suggests true cephalopelvic disproportion.

If the position of the head is occipito-posterior, the station of the head will determine whether a vaginal delivery is possible. This can either be performed with rotational forceps, e.g. Kjellands or vacuum extractor (see Ch. 27), or with lift-out forceps if the head is low enough.

Cephalo-pelvic disproportion

This term is used only in the context of primigravidae. In the past, slow progress in the first stage of labour was wrongly termed cephalo-pelvic disproportion, whereas now the most likely diagnosis is considered to be inefficient uterine action and this is treated with an oxytocin infusion.

If progress still fails to occur, then a tentative diagnosis of cephalo-pelvic disproportion can be entertained, provided the head is not occipito-posterior. If these strict criteria are applied to make the diagnosis, one in 250 primigravidae will have cephalo-pelvic disproportion, and if allowed to labour subsequently, 50% will deliver vaginally.

True cephalo-pelvic disproportion is rare, and the diagnosis can only be made in retrospect. Once this diagnosis has been made it will strongly influence the mode of delivery in subsequent pregnancies.

Parous women: cephalopelvic disproportion can occur due to either a larger fetus, or a reduction in pelvic capacity, or both. The uterine action in these cases will be vigorously reactive and the risk of uterine rupture is considerable, especially if oxytocin is used. The diagnosis rests on features such as delay in descent of the presenting part, exaggerated moulding and unremitting uterine activity.

SUMMARY

A prolonged second stage of labour requires sensible management if maternal and fetal trauma are to be avoided.

25. Labour—third stage

J. Rymer

Expectations of the examiners

A thorough knowledge of the normal and abnormal third stage is essential. The candidate should appreciate that proper management of the third stage is of vital importance in reducing the incidence of postpartum haemorrhage, retained placenta, and consequent maternal morbidity and mortality.

Definition

The third stage commences with the delivery of the baby and finishes with delivery of the placenta.

Interesting facts

Postpartum haemorrhage is the most common cause of serious blood loss in obstetrics. It is an important cause of maternal mortality, accounting for 33% of maternal deaths from haemorrhage in England and Wales. (Report on Confidential Enquiries into Maternal Deaths 1982–1984.)

Physiology

The continuation of uterine contractions, and the reduction of surface area of the uterine cavity cause the placenta to separate from the uterine wall. As separation occurs there is some retroplacental bleeding which contributes to the separation process.

There are two processes which help to control excessive bleeding from the placental bed:

1. The interlacing bundles of muscle in the uterine wall contract and twist compressing the vessels as the uterus decreases in size.
2. Normal coagulation, i.e. release of thromboplastins, platelet aggregation, and fibrin formation.

Table 25.1 Risk factors for postpartum haem-orrhage.

Past history of a postpartum haemorrhage
Grand multiparity
Uterine overdistension (e.g. large baby, twins)
Antepartum haemorrhage
Coagulation disorders
Poor uterine contractions
Prolonged labour
Large placental bed (e.g. rhesus disease)
Operative delivery

Haemostatic processes may be less efficient in the following circumstances:

1. Dysfunctional labour
2. Uterine overdistension, e.g. multiple pregnancy
3. Anaesthetic agents, e.g. halothane
4. Morbid adherence of the placenta.

Assessment

Risk factors for a postpartum haemorrhage should be identified in the patient's previous obstetric history (see Table 25.1) or current pregnancy.

Management

The policy for management of the third stage varies between obstetric units. As the anterior shoulder is delivered an ecbolic is administered i.m. or i.v. in the form of oxytocin ± ergometrine (see Table 25.2). The placenta is usually delivered by the Brandt–Andrews technique. The cord is held with the right hand and downward traction is applied while the uterus is lifted upwards with the left hand placed suprapubically. If the placenta does not advance then it is usually still attached to the uterus. If the placenta is not delivered after 30 minutes then a manual removal is required (see Complications). Once the placenta has been delivered the fundus is briefly massaged to ensure that it contracts. The genital tract must be

Table 25.2 Time from administration to action on the uterus for the various oxytocic drugs.

Drug	Administration	Time
Oxytocin	i.v.	30 seconds
Ergometrine	i.v.	40 seconds
Oxytocin	i.m.	2.5 minutes
Ergometrine + oxytocin	i.m.	2.5 minutes
Ergometrine	i.m.	7 minutes

inspected for any lacerations and repaired appropriately. The placenta should be examined to ensure completeness and normality.

An assessment of the blood loss should be recorded.

Complications

Postpartum haemorrhage

A primary postpartum haemorrhage is defined as a blood loss $\geqslant 500\,\mathrm{ml}$ within 24 hours of delivery. The incidence of postpartum haemorrhage is 5% of deliveries.

Aetiology

1. Uterine atony
2. Local trauma to vagina or cervix
3. Retained placenta or products of conception
4. Other:
   a. Uterine inversion
   b. Uterine rupture
   c. Defective coagulation.

Management. The assessment and treatment should take place simultaneously.

Examine the fundus. If it is high and soft then uterine atony and/or retained products are the cause of the bleeding. The fundus should be massaged to expel clot and ensure maximum retraction. In severe haemorrhage, bimanual compression with the uterus compressed between a vaginal and an abdominal hand can be used. If the fundus is not palpable then uterine inversion should be suspected and an immediate vaginal examination performed. The placenta and membranes should be checked to ensure they are complete.

Resuscitation. An i.v. line of large bore (14 g or greater) should be inserted while the initial examination is taking place (two lines in severe cases). Blood should be sent for FBC, clotting studies and four units of whole blood crossmatched. Initially, crystalloid or plasma substitute should be infused as quickly as required.

Examination of the genital tract. If the fundus is retracted and bleeding is continuing then careful speculum examination should be carried out and vaginal or cervical lacerations repaired appropriately.

Further measures. Further management depends on the findings and response to the measures already mentioned.

1. Uterine atony. In most cases this will respond to massage and the bleeding will settle. A syntocinon infusion should be commenced (40 U syntocinon in 500 ml of crystalloid over 2–4 hours) or ergometrine 0.5 mg i.m. can be given if the patient has no history of cardiac disease or

hypertension at any stage in pregnancy. If these measures are not successful, the uterine cavity should be examined under general anaesthesia (or epidural if one is already in situ) to remove any retained products. If bleeding continues, then prostaglandin injected directly into the myometrium is usually effective but, if not, then surgery should be performed without delay. Internal iliac artery ligation is often discussed but may not effectively control bleeding and hysterectomy should be undertaken sooner rather than later.

2. Retained products/placenta should be removed with great care under anaesthesia. It is important that maximum uterine retraction is maintained until removal and this is best accomplished by syntocinon infusion and fundal massage if necessary.

3. Uterine rupture. If an EUA reveals a hole in the uterus then a laparotomy must be performed. If possible the tear is repaired, but if haemostasis cannot be achieved then a postpartum hysterectomy or internal iliac ligation (or embolization) can be performed.

Retained placenta

If the placenta is not delivered within 30 minutes then preparations should be made for a manual removal. This can be performed under spinal, epidural, or general anaesthesia.

Uterine inversion

The fundus of the uterus descends through the cervix usually with the placenta still attached. This has become a rare complication with the use of oxytocics and the Brandt–Andrews technique. Management involves immediate reduction if possible. If this is ineffective, then an i.v. line must be inserted, blood crossmatched, and the hydrostatic method of reduction attempted. Sterile saline is run into the upper vagina while the forearm occludes the introitus. If this fails, then abdominal surgery is required.

Amniotic fluid embolism

The patient suddenly collapses and a severe coagulation defect develops. If recognized, the patient needs to be ventilated, given steroids, and the coagulation defect corrected. The diagnosis is usually made at post mortem.

26. Fetal monitoring in labour

J. Rymer

Interesting facts

The aim of fetal monitoring in labour is to detect fetal hypoxia so that resulting perinatal morbidity and mortality can be prevented. The reaction of the fetus to hypoxia is variable and dependent on its individual reserve. Therefore each fetus should be assessed for its relative risk of developing hypoxia in labour and surveillance during labour managed accordingly.

Methods

There are various methods of monitoring a fetus during labour:

Note the colour of the liquor. Meconium staining may result from an episode of hypoxia which causes vagal stimulation of the gut, relaxing the anal sphincter. Thick fresh meconium is considered an ominous sign. The absence of liquor is associated with IUGR and the fetus should be treated as if the liquor is meconium-stained until proven otherwise.

Auscultation of the fetal heart using a Pinard's stethoscope. This is an intermittent form of fetal monitoring and should be employed during and immediately after contractions to detect accelerations or decelerations in the fetal heart rate. It is useful in low-risk patients with no identifiable abnormalities.

Sonar pulse detector (sonicaid). This is also an intermittent form of fetal monitoring and should be used in a similar way to the Pinard stethoscope.

Continuous fetal heart rate monitoring. This method involves either an abdominal transducer, which detects the fetal heart movements ultrasonically, or an electrode attached to the fetal scalp which records a signal from the fetal heart (Fig. 26.1). The abdominal transducer is less accurate. Most recording instruments also record uterine activity.

Fetal heart rate patterns

Normal. The normal baseline heart rate is between 120–160 beats/minute. Brief accelerations of 10–15 beats/minute indicate a healthy fetus.

a

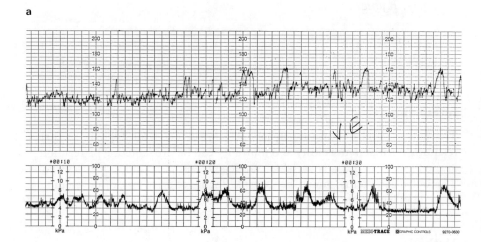

b

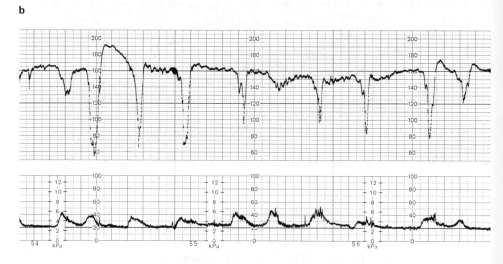

Fig. 26.1 Cardiotocographs (CTGs). **a**. Normal reactive trace; **b**. early decelerations.

Baseline variability should be 5–15 beats/minute and beat to beat variability 3–5 beats.

Baseline tachycardia. (FHR > 160/minute.) Associated with certain drugs, prematurity, hypoxia, or maternal pyrexia.

Baseline bradycardia. (FHR < 120/minute.) Between 90–120 is only significant if there are decelerations or decreased variability. It may be rarely due to congenital heart block. Severe bradycardia (< 90 beats/minute) is usually associated with a preterminal condition in the fetus.

Loss of baseline variability. A normal heart rate shows irregular accelerations and if this variation is lost it may indicate chronic hypoxia.

Early decelerations (Fig. 26.2). These decelerations begin with the onset of a contraction and return to the baseline by the end of the contraction. They are usually due to compression of the fetal head and are not a sign of fetal distress.

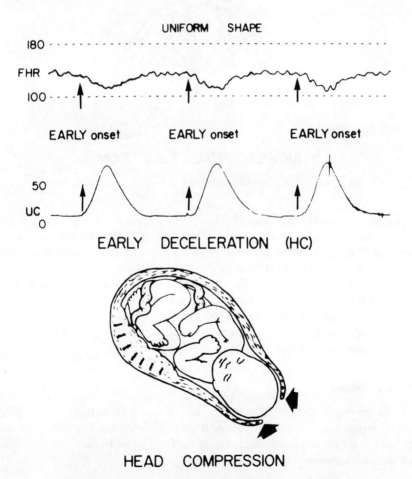

Fig. 26.2   Head compression and early deceleration (HC).

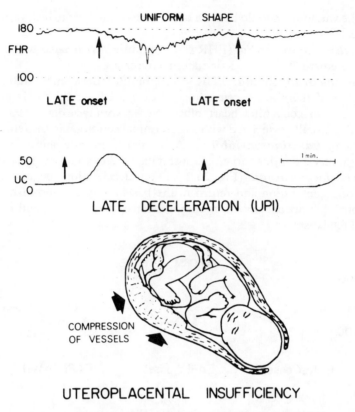

Fig. 26.3 Uteroplacental insufficiency and late deceleration (UPI).

Late decelerations (Fig. 26.3). The low point of the deceleration occurs after the peak of the contraction and the fetal heart rate is slow to recover. The greater the lag-time between the end of the contraction and the return of the fetal heart rate to its normal baseline, the more serious is the hypoxia likely to be. Late decelerations are usually associated with fetal hypoxia and fetal blood sampling is indicated if labour is to proceed.

Variable decelerations (Fig. 26.4). These include all other decelerations and their interpretation is difficult. They may be associated with cord compression.

Management

In the low-risk mother it is acceptable to use intermittent monitoring. Interpreting continuous FHR recordings is difficult and the whole clinical picture must be taken into account. If the fetal heart tracing suggests fetal distress then various steps can be taken:

1. Delivery, e.g. if a woman is in early labour with thick meconium-stained

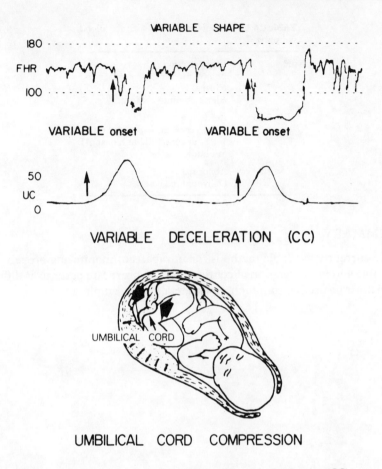

VARIABLE   SHAPE

VARIABLE onset   VARIABLE onset

VARIABLE   DECELERATION   (CC)

UMBILICAL   CORD

UMBILICAL   CORD   COMPRESSION

Fig. 26.4 Umbilical cord compression and variable deceleration (CC).

liquor and there are persistent late decelerations, then abdominal delivery is advised.
2. Fetal blood sampling. This should be regarded as complementary to continuous FHR recording. If the latter facility is used alone then the caesarean section rate will be higher due to false positive diagnoses (see Table 26.1).
3. Resuscitation. If the cause of acute fetal distress is due to a correctable maternal condition, then appropriate measures should be undertaken.
    a. The patient should adopt a lateral position with the foot of the bed higher than her heart.
    b. Augmentation should be discontinued and in rare cases, uterine action should be inhibited using a tocolytic drug.
    c. Maternal hypotension should be corrected.
    d. The mother should be given oxygen.

Table 26.1 Interpretation of fetal blood sampling.

pH	Interpretation
> 7.25	Normal Allow labour to continue
7.20–7.25	Borderline If delivery is anticipated within 1–2 hours proceed but repeat pH in 1 hour
< 7.20	Abnormal Deliver immediately

SUMMARY

The currently available methods for intrapartum monitoring are still unreliable and interpretation of continuous fetal heart rate patterns is difficult and must be used in conjunction with fetal blood sampling.

27. Obstetric intervention

J. Rymer

INDUCTION OF LABOUR

Expectations of the examiners

The candidate should be familiar with the common indications and current methods of induction.

Interesting facts

Historically, induction of labour was mainly performed to ensure a small baby in cases of severe pelvic deformity.

Indications

Labour can be induced for numerous maternal and/or fetal reasons. When considering induction, two factors must be considered: 1. the risk to the mother or fetus if the pregnancy continues, vs. 2. the risk of preterm delivery and complications of induction. The absolute contraindications are:

1. Placenta praevia
2. Abnormal lie
3. Known cephalo-pelvic disproportion.

Assessment

Important factors that must be considered prior to induction of labour are:

1. Gestation
2. Maternal well-being
3. Fetal well-being.

In order to determine the method of induction the maternal abdomen must be palpated noting the presentation of the fetus, and whether the head is engaged or unengaged. A vaginal examination should be performed. The consistency, position, length, and dilatation of the cervix should be

Table 27.1　Bishop's score (inducibility rating).

Dilatation	0	1–2	3–4	5–6
Score	0	1	2	3
Length of the cervix (cm)	3	2	1	0
Score	0	1	2	3
Station	−3	−2	−1 0	+1 +2
Score	0	1	2	3
Consistency	Firm	Medium	Soft	
Score	0	1	2	
Position	Posterior	Mid	Anterior	
Score	0	1	2	

Total score = 0–5 unfavourable
6–13 favourable

documented and the station of the presenting part. (See Bishop's score, Table 27.1.) If the cervix is unfavourable the chances of a good response to labour induction are low.

Method

If the presenting part is not high and an artificial rupture of membranes (ARM) is technically possible, then the patient should be transferred to the labour ward, and an ARM performed under aseptic conditions. This can be performed with an amnihook or Kocher's forceps, and after the membranes have been ruptured, they should be swept back to release further prostaglandins. Some patients will spontaneously commence labour if left alone, but the majority require augmentation. A syntocinon infusion is used, either immediately or after a period of time, initially at a low dose, and increasing every 15 minutes, until regular contractions are established. The fetal heart rate must be monitored; in most centres this is done continuously, and the cervical dilatation should be assessed regularly.

If the cervix is unfavourable, then prostaglandins can be used. The current trend is to use intravaginal preparations, e.g. pessaries or gel. The state of the cervix is reassessed after an interval, and if possible the membranes are ruptured. If the cervix remains unfavourable, a further dose of prostaglandin can be used. The dosage and timing of prostaglandin administration is very variable.

Complications of induction

1. Fetal distress
2. Maternal distress
3. Precipitate delivery
4. Operative delivery

5. Iatrogenic prematurity
6. Uterine rupture
7. Amniotic fluid embolism
8. Water intoxication (if high doses of syntocinon and too much fluid)
9. Diarrhoea, nausea, vomiting (systemic effects of prostaglandins).

SUMMARY

Induced labours have a higher incidence of operative deliveries, and the recent trend has been away from induction. The decision for induction must include the consideration of risks and benefits to both mother and fetus.

FORCEPS DELIVERIES

Expectations of the examiners

The candidate should be familiar with nonrotational forceps, e.g. Wrigley's and Neville Barnes', and be able to discuss the indications and prerequisites for forceps delivery. The candidate should also have a basic understanding of Kjelland's forceps but would not be expected to use these rotational forceps.

Interesting facts

A pair of forceps consists of two instruments, each a mirror image of the other. There are four components: a blade, a shank, a lock, and a handle. Each blade has a cephalic and a pelvic curve (Figs 27.1–27.2).

Indications for use

There must be a maternal and/or fetal reason to expedite delivery:

1. Fetal
   a. Distress
   b. Aftercoming head of breech
2. Maternal
   a. Delay in second stage
   b. Maternal disease, e.g. cardiac disease
   c. Dural tap.

Assessment

The following requirements must be satisfied before a forceps delivery can be performed:

1. Adequate analgesia

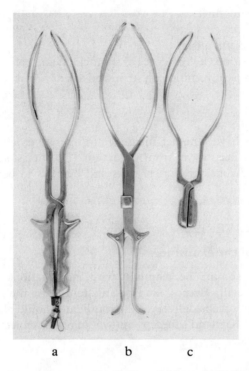

                    a   b   c

Fig. 27.1   Forceps in common use. **a**. Neville Barnes' forceps; **b**. Kjelland's forceps; **c**. Wrigley's forceps.

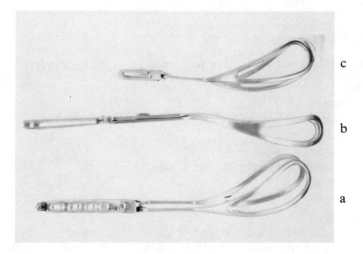

Fig. 27.2   Lateral view of the forceps shown in Fig. 27.1 reveals that the Wrigley and the Neville–Barnes forceps have a much larger pelvic curve than the Kjelland forceps (middle pair).

2. Bladder empty
3. No obvious cephalo-pelvic disproportion present
4. Cervix must be fully dilated
5. There must be no head palpable above the pelvic brim
6. The membranes must not be intact
7. The position of the fetal head must be known, i.e. occipito-anterior $\pm$ 15
8. The head must be at station $+2$ or more.

Method

The patient is placed in the lithotomy position and cleaned and draped. The bladder is emptied, and local anaesthesia is injected at this point if it is the chosen method of analgesia. The position and station of the vertex is checked. The left blade is applied first, followed by the right, and they should lock together easily if the application is correct. The direction of traction is initially forward and down, following the normal axis of delivery (only 3 pulls are allowed). As the perineum becomes distended, the head is extended, and an episiotomy is usually performed. The forceps are removed, and the delivery is conducted as normal. After delivery of the placenta, the perineum and vaginal walls are inspected, and any tears appropriately repaired.

Rotational forceps

Kjelland's forceps have a cephalic curve, but no pelvic curve, and a sliding lock to correct for asynclitism. They are used when rotation of the head is required and should only be used by experienced obstetricians as they can cause significant maternal and fetal injury.

Complications

1. Fetal. Incorrect application of the forceps has been implicated in intra-cranial haemorrhage, and direct damage to the facial structures can occur (e.g. eye, nose).
2. Maternal. Trauma to the birth canal is common and uterine rupture can occur. Postpartum haemorrhage is more common due to genital tract trauma and prolonged and difficult labour.

VENTOUSE DELIVERIES

Expectations of the examiners

The candidate is expected to be able to recognize the instrument and understand the principles behind its use.

Definition

A vacuum extractor (Ventouse) is a suction cap connected to a suction device. A vacuum is created between the cap and the fetal scalp and traction is applied in the axis of the birth canal to expedite delivery.

Indications for use

The indications are the same as for forceps deliveries, but maternal effort is needed. Therefore, in situations where maternal effort must be avoided, e.g. cardiac disease, severe hypertension, the Ventouse is contraindicated.

An incompletely dilated cervix is not an indication in modern obstetrics.

Requirements for a Ventouse delivery

The same as for a forceps delivery.

Method

The patient is prepared as for a forceps delivery. The cup is placed over the posterior fontanelle, and a vacuum of $0.8\,kg/cm^2$ is created. Traction is applied in the axis of the birth canal, imitating the normal mechanism of labour. Delivery must occur within three pulls, as with forceps deliveries.

Complications

Mainly fetal scalp injuries.

1. Cephalhaematoma—bleeding beneath the periosteum
2. Subgaleal haematoma—bleeding beneath the galea caused by emissary vein rupture
3. Intracranial haemorrhage—this complication is rare and related to hypoxia and prematurity.

These can be avoided if the technique is used appropriately.

The Ventouse has specific advantages over the forceps:

1. It can be used with minimal or no anaesthesia
2. It occupies no space between the fetal head and the maternal tissues
3. There is less risk of maternal and fetal injury if used correctly.

CAESAREAN SECTION

Expectations of the examiners

The examiners will assume that the candidate has assisted at caesarean sections. The indications, risks, and complications of the operation should be known and the management of future deliveries. The caesarean section rate at the candidate's hospital should be known.

Definition

A caesarean section is a surgical procedure whereby the fetus is delivered abdominally through a uterine incision.

Interesting facts

Although low, the maternal mortality following caesarean section is significantly greater than the maternal mortality following vaginal delivery. A woman's obstetric future may be prejudiced by the presence of a uterine scar.

Indications

There are many indications for caesarean section and the commonest are listed below:

1. Fetal
   a. Fetal distress—this can either be antenatally or intrapartum
   b. Malpresentations and malpositions
   c. Multiple pregnancy
2. Maternal
   a. Failure to progress in labour
   b. Previous caesarean section—most obstetricians would deliver a woman who had had two previous caesarean sections by an elective caesarean section
   c. Pre-eclampsia or eclampsia
   d. Cephalo-pelvic disproportion
3. Placental
   a. Praevia
   b. Abruption
   c. Cord prolapse.

With most of the indications listed above, other factors may need to be taken into account, e.g. gestation, stage of labour, parity.

Method

The operation can be performed under epidural, general, or spinal anaesthesia. The bladder is emptied and the woman is placed in the left lateral position to avoid supine hypotension. The abdomen is cleaned and draped. Most caesarean sections are performed through a horizontal suprapubic skin incision (Pfannenstiel). The various layers of the abdominal wall are divided to expose the lower segment of the uterus. A transverse incision is made in the lower segment and the presenting part is then delivered manually or with forceps (if cephalic), the baby's mouth is suctioned, and the rest of the body is extracted. The cord is clamped and cut, and the placenta is removed. The wound is then repaired in layers.

A 'classical' caesarean section involves a vertical skin incision (although it can be done through a lower suprapubic skin incision) and a vertical incision in the upper segment of the uterus. This leaves a large scar on the uterus which is weaker in subsequent pregnancies. Most obstetricians would deliver a woman who had had a classical caesarean with an elective caesarean in subsequent pregnancies.

Requirements

1. Ideally the patient should be starved and given a H2 antagonist and an alkaline mixture prior to the operation (to neutralize the acid in the stomach)
2. The bladder must be empty
3. An intravenous line must be in place
4. An experienced anaesthetist must be present
5. Blood must be available.

Complications

Early

1. Anaesthetic problems, e.g. failed intubation, drug overdose, hypoxia, aspiration of gastric contents
2. Haemorrhage
3. Bladder and bowel damage
4. The original condition that caused the operation, e.g. pre-eclampsia may worsen postoperatively.

Late

1. Infection, e.g. uterine, wound, chest
2. Thromboembolism
3. Haemorrhage
4. Urinary tract infection
5. Wound dehiscence
6. Psychological problems.

Very late

1. Infertility (following infection)
2. Uterine rupture in a subsequent pregnancy
3. Adhesion formation.

SUMMARY

The maternal morbidity and mortality for a caesarean section are higher when compared with a vaginal delivery.

28. Breech presentation and transverse lie

J. Rymer

BREECH PRESENTATION

Expectations of the examiners

Although the delivery of a breech presentation is a specialist area, the examiners will expect the candidate to understand the principles of antenatal and labour management. As a general practitioner, the candidate may well have to perform a breech delivery if it has not been diagnosed prior to delivery, or there is not enough time to call the flying squad as in preterm labour. There are several areas of controversy in the management of breech presentation, and the candidate could be expected to discuss these.

Definition

The word breech means 'the buttocks'. There are three types of breech:

1. Extended leg breech—the legs are flexed at the hip and extended at the knee (frank breech).
2. Flexed leg breech—the legs are flexed at the hip and the knee (complete).
3. Footling breech—one or both feet are below the buttocks.

Interesting facts

The incidence is 3–4% of all singleton pregnancies. The morbidity and mortality for a fetus in a breech presentation are considerably worse than for a vertex presentation. (Major contributors to this are prematurity, congenital anomalies and birth trauma.)

Aetiology

1. Maternal
   a. Grand multiparity
   b. Uterine anomalies
   c. Pelvic tumours
   d. Bony pelvic abnormality.

2. Fetal
   a. Prematurity
   b. Multiple pregnancy
   c. Fetal abnormality
   d. Extended legs.
3. Placental
   a. Cornual implantation
   b. Placenta praevia
   c. Oligohydramnios
   d. Polyhydramnios.

Assessment

The frequency of breech presentation decreases as pregnancy progresses. A breech presentation does not become a concern until 36 weeks (except in preterm labour). External cephalic version used to be performed between 32 and 36 weeks to convert the breech to a cephalic presentation. It is a hazardous procedure and is now not recommended.

The diagnosis of a breech presentation is made on palpation of the abdomen. The presenting part is wider and the head is felt in the fundus. The fetal heart is heard above the umbilicus.

If the position of the placenta is known, then a vaginal examination should be performed to exclude pelvic masses and gross abnormalities of the pelvic bones.

Investigations

An ultrasound scan should be performed for the following reasons:

1. To confirm presentation
2. To exclude a fetal abnormality
3. To determine placental position
4. To determine whether it is a flexed or extended leg breech
5. To assess the liquor volume
6. To estimate fetal weight.

X-ray pelvimetry is performed to exclude pelvic abnormality. The antero-posterior diameter of the pelvic inlet should be greater than 11.5 cm.

Management

Once ultrasound scan and pelvimetry have been performed, a decision on the mode of delivery should be made. The ideal weight for a vaginal breech delivery is 2500–3500 g. Footling and flexed leg breeches are usually delivered by caesarean section but in a multiparous woman a flexed leg breech may be allowed a trial of labour. Providing there are no maternal contraindications, an extended leg breech, without a fetal abnormality, between 2500–3500 g is favourable for a trial of vaginal delivery.

Most practitioners would not induce a breech presentation as spontaneous onset of labour has the best prognosis. Once labour is established the membranes should be ruptured, and a fetal scalp electrode applied to the buttock. An epidural anaesthetic is ideal because of the need for an operative delivery. The fetus should be monitored continuously and progress in labour assessed regularly. The use of syntocinon augmentation in a breech presentation is controversial, and slow progress in labour (< 1 cm/h) is usually managed by a caesarean section.

Once full dilatation has occurred and the breech has descended to the perineum then an episiotomy should be performed. As the breech continues to descend the sacrum is gently guided anteriorly, and the legs are stepped over the perineum (Pinard's manoeuvre). As the trunk descends the shoulders are delivered. If there is difficulty in delivering the shoulders then Lovset's manoeuvre must be performed. (Lovset's manoeuvre involves rotating the posterior shoulder anteriorly by rotating the trunk and then applying a downward traction. This enables the shoulders to descend below the pelvic rim and the arm usually appears spontaneously. If not, a finger can be hooked over the anterior shoulder and the arm brought down. The manoeuvre is repeated for the other arm.) The baby is allowed to hang until the nape of the neck is visible. The assistant then lifts the baby up and forceps are applied to the head to ensure a controlled delivery.

SUMMARY

Breech presentation is associated with increased perinatal morbidity and mortality, and must be considered a high-risk pregnancy.

TRANSVERSE AND OBLIQUE LIE

Expectations of the examiners

The candidate should be able to detect abnormal lie on palpation. The principles of management of a transverse and oblique lie should be known by the candidate. The management of cord prolapse is a common examination question

Definition

The lie of the fetus is not in the longitudinal axis of the uterus.

Aetiology

1. Maternal
   a. High multiparity
   b. Uterine anomalies
   c. Pelvic tumours
   d. Pelvic contraction
2. Fetal
   a. Prematurity
   b. Multiple pregnancy
   c. Fetal abnormality
3. Placenta
   a. Placenta praevia
   b. Fundal placenta.

Assessment

On inspection the uterus appears wider than normal. The fundal height may be smaller than one would expect for the gestational age, and there is no presenting part in the pelvis. The back is lying across the maternal abdomen and the head is palpated in one or other flank. The fetal heart may be heard more laterally than normal.

As with a breech presentation, a vaginal examination should be performed (if the placental site is known) to exclude pelvic pathology.

Investigations

An ultrasound scan should be performed for the same reasons as in breech presentation.

Management

Transverse lie is uncommon. External cephalic version should not be attempted. If the transverse lie persists beyond 37 weeks then the woman should be admitted to hospital, because of the risk of cord prolapse. If a cause for the transverse lie is found, e.g. pelvic tumour, placenta praevia, then an elective caesarean section should be performed. If no cause is found then there are two accepted forms of management:

1. Await the onset of labour to see if the lie converts to longitudinal in labour. If it does, then the woman has a trial of labour. If it does not, then a caesarean section should be performed. If the lie converts to longitudinal prior to the onset of labour she can be allowed home. In primiparous women this is very unlikely after 37 weeks, even when labour begins.
2. An elective caesarean section can be performed.

Cord prolapse

If a woman with a transverse lie has spontaneous rupture of membranes she must have an immediate vaginal examination to exclude cord prolapse. If the cord is felt then the woman must be put into the knee–chest position, or placed on all fours. The aim of adopting these positions is to use gravity to keep the presenting part from compressing the cord against the cervix. The examining hand must remain in the vagina to elevate the presenting part until the baby is delivered. (If there is to be a long delay between the time of cord prolapse and caesarean section then 500 ml of fluid can be infused into the bladder via a Foley catheter which is then clamped.)

Urgent arrangements must be made to deliver the baby by caesarean section.

Delivery

A transverse lie that persists must be delivered by caesarean section. These can be difficult operations, especially if the fetal back is presenting.

A general anaesthetic is preferred to ensure the maximum uterine relaxation. If there is no lower segment then a vertical incision should be performed in the uterus. After incising the uterus, a breech extraction is performed. A foot is grasped, the lie converted to longitudinal, and the feet and the remainder of the body are delivered.

A thorough inspection of the uterine cavity and the pelvis should be performed to attempt to determine a cause for the transverse lie.

SUMMARY

Transverse and oblique lie is uncommon and needs specialist referral. Women should be admitted from 37 weeks onwards. Cord prolapse is more common and is an obstetric emergency.

29. Twin pregnancy

J. Rymer

Expectations of the examiners

The candidate will be expected to be aware of the common antenatal complications of a multiple pregnancy. The overall management of multiple pregnancy should always be undertaken by a specialist unit.

Definition

A pregnancy with two fetuses.

Interesting facts

The incidence is 1 in 80 but this is increasing due to assisted conception techniques.

Pathophysiology

Twinning can either be monozygotic or dizygotic. Monozygotic twins result from the division of one conceptus, producing identical twins. Dizygotic twins result from the fertilization of two separate ova, and the twins have different genetic make-up. Dizygotic twins are always dichorionic and diamniotic, but monozygotic twins can vary from monochorionic and monoamniotic to dichorionic and diamniotic, depending on when division of the blastocyst occurred.

Aetiology

The frequency of monozygotic twins is constant at a rate of one set/250 births. However, the incidence of dizygotic twins is influenced remarkably by:

1. Race. In Nigeria twinning occurs 1 in every 19 births, compared to 1 in 155 births in Japan.
2. Heredity. A family history of twins, especially on the mother's side, is associated with an increase in the incidence of twin pregnancy.

3. Increasing maternal age and parity. Both of these factors are associated with a higher rate of twin pregnancies.
4. Assisted conception. The overall incidence of multiple pregnancies using these techniques is 2–3%. This is due to the induction of multiple ovulations and the replacement of more than one egg or embryo.

Assessment

At the booking visit, the history may include risk factors for multiple pregnancy as outlined above. 'Hyperemesis gravidarum' in the first trimester is more common, and on examination the uterine size may be larger than dates.

Investigations

An ultrasound scan should detect multiple pregnancies, although they can be missed.

The haemoglobin and the packed cell volume may be lower due to the exaggerated increase in plasma volume.

The alpha fetoprotein levels in maternal serum will be higher, making interpretation difficult.

Management

Multiple pregnancy should not be regarded as a 'normal pregnancy', and patients should be seen more regularly in the antenatal clinic.

First trimester. An early scan (< 14 weeks) should be performed for dating purposes. Severe hyperemesis warrants admission with intravenous hydration. Four weekly visits are acceptable if there are no other complications.

Second trimester. A detailed anomaly scan should be performed at 16–18 weeks as there is an increased incidence of fetal abnormalities.

Third trimester. After 28 weeks' gestation the patient should be seen at least twice weekly with regular ultrasound scans for growth assessment.

Routine admission at 28 weeks to 32 weeks has not been shown to decrease the incidence of premature labour. Admission should be offered to the patient at any stage if she is unable to rest adequately at home.

In late pregnancy the commonest presentations are vertex, vertex (45%); vertex, breech (40%); but malpresentations are more common in multiple pregnancies.

Complications

Maternal

1. Hyperemesis. Severe cases require admission and intravenous

hydration, but most settle by 12 weeks when the beta HCG levels begin to fall.

2. Hypertension. Not only does hypertension occur more often in multiple pregnancy but it tends to develop earlier, and be more severe.
3. Gestational diabetes. The diabetogenic state of normal pregnancy is exaggerated, increasing the incidence and severity of gestational diabetes.
4. Anaemia. The increase in plasma volume is much greater, exaggerating the 'physiological' anaemia of pregnancy. Iron and folate deficiencies are common because of the extra demands of a twin pregnancy.
5. General discomfort. Having a larger uterine mass puts added strain on the musculoskeletal system.
6. Placenta praevia. The incidence is increased in multiple pregnancies presumably due to the increased placental area.

Fetal

1. Prematurity is the main factor in the increased wastage associated with multiple pregnancies. More than 50% of babies of multiple pregnancies are less than 2.5 kg compared with 6% of singletons. There are many contributing factors to the significantly increased incidence of preterm delivery in twin pregnancies:
   a. Overdistension of the uterus
   b. Increased incidence of pregnancy induced hypertension
   c. Increased incidence of fetal abnormalities
   d. Increased incidence of abruption
   e. Increased incidence of malpresentation.
2. Fetal abnormality. There is an increased incidence of fetal malformation in monozygotic twin pregnancies.
3. IUGR. Growth retardation is common in twin pregnancies especially when the placenta is monochorionic. One or both twins may be affected.
4. Twin-to-twin transfusion. The two placental circulations may form anastomoses in monochorionic twins. One fetus may become anaemic, and the other polycythaemic. The syndrome is usually diagnosed after birth, and either baby may require intensive care.
5. Malpresentations. Probably more common because of prematurity, increased incidence of fetal malformations, and mechanical restrictions of the uterine cavity.

Delivery

The decision on the mode of delivery depends on the presentation of the leading twin, and the presence of maternal or fetal complications. In the majority of cases, labour occurs spontaneously around 38 weeks.

The membranes should be ruptured as soon as labour is established. An intravenous line should be inserted, and blood should be grouped and saved. A fetal scalp electrode should be applied to the leading twin, and the second twin monitored externally.

An epidural is the optimal form of analgesia, as an operative delivery may be required.

Progress in labour must be assessed regularly as inefficient uterine action is common.

At delivery, two obstetricians, two paediatricians, an anaesthetist and midwifery staff should be present. Following delivery of the first twin, the cord is clamped and cut. The abdomen is palpated to ensure that the lie of the remaining fetus is longitudinal. (If the lie cannot be converted to longitudinal externally, then a caesarean section should be considered.) Fundal pressure is maintained, and the membranes ruptured during a contraction. Labour should resume, but if there are no contractions after 10 minutes, then a syntocinon infusion should be commenced. The second twin is then delivered. Breech extraction of the second twin may be necessary. The placenta is delivered, and a syntocinon infusion postpartum is advisable to prevent haemorrhage.

Complications

1. Incoordinate uterine action. This is a common occurrence in twins. There is debate as to whether labour should be augmented.
2. Fetal distress. The second twin is usually smaller and may not cope as well with the stress of labour.
3. Prolapse of the umbilical cord. The management depends on the circumstances: degree of cervical dilatation, the presence or absence of ruptured membranes, and the analgesia. (see Ch. 28.)
4. Premature separation of the placenta. If vaginal delivery can be achieved rapidly without harm to the fetus or the mother, then this should be performed. Otherwise, the fetus should be delivered by caesarean section.
5. Locking. This is rare but can occur when the first twin presents as a breech, and the second by the vertex. The chin of the first fetus locks in the neck and chin of the second cephalic fetus.

Postpartum

1. Haemorrhage. Due to the increased size of the placental bed, and the overdistension of the uterus, there is an increased risk of postpartum haemorrhage.
2. Thromboembolic disease. Twin pregnancies have an increased risk.
3. Anaemia. Due to the increased demand for iron in pregnancy and the greater blood loss.

SUMMARY

Twin pregnancies have significantly increased fetal and maternal morbidity and mortality. They are high-risk pregnancies and should be monitored carefully. The delivery should be conducted in a specialist unit. Only twin pregnancies have been discussed but the problems of a twin gestation are exaggerated by the presence of more fetuses. Most obstetricians would deliver pregnancies with three or more fetuses by caesarean section.

30. Obstetric analgesia and anaesthesia

G. Davis

Expectations of the examiners

Candidates will be expected to know and be able to advise on the relative merits of the different methods of analgesia and anaesthesia. An understanding of the importance of effects on mother and fetus and the complications and their management is required.

Definitions

Analgesia: loss of sensation to pain.
Anaesthesia: loss of all sensation including pain.

Interesting facts

There is a wide range of methods available for pain relief and the choice of any method will depend on a number of factors: mother's preference, severity of pain, stage in labour, methods available and any complications in the mother and/or fetus. Anxiety is a significant component of labour for most women and their partners. Careful explanation and reassurance to reduce anxiety is an important aspect of the management of pain in labour. Patients vary widely in their tolerance of pain and their response to analgesia.

Pathophysiology

Source of the pain: pain in labour is of two types: 1. intermittent, and 2. continuous.

Intermittent pain is due to uterine contractions and is probably due to myometrial ischaemia at the peak of the contractions. The pain is most severe just prior to full dilatation (transition phase) when contractions are most intense and the cervix is dilating most rapidly. Sensation from the uterus and cervix is transmitted mainly in the sensory fibres of the T11 and T12 nerve roots with smaller amounts in T10 and L1.

Continuous pain occurs in the lower back and suprapubically and the cause of this pain is not known. Lower back pain is more prominent with occipito-posterior positions.

In the second stage of labour, pain is associated with distension of the lower vagina and perineum. The perineum is innervated principally by the pudendal nerve (posterior two-thirds of vulva) with fibres passing to S2, 3 and 4.

Pharmacokinetics in mother and fetus

Mother. Although liver production of various proteins alters markedly in pregnancy, it is unclear whether this affects the maternal handling of anaesthetic drugs in any way. Body fat stores increase by 4 kg on average during pregnancy leading to a greater capacity to sequester lipid-soluble drugs.

Fetus. About one-seventh of the blood returning to the fetus from the placenta enters the left atrium directly. Any drugs in this blood are therefore available to affect the fetal brain. This is only likely to be significant with intravenous bolus injections and conversely six-sevenths of the umbilical blood flow passes through the fetal liver where drugs will be metabolized.

Placental transfer

Like the blood–brain barrier, the placental barrier is composed of lipo-proteins so the transfer of drugs will depend on lipid solubility. Most agents which affect the central nervous system will therefore cross the placenta. Highly ionized drugs, such as muscle relaxants, do not cross the placenta.

Although there has been concern that exposure of pregnant women to trace quantities of anaesthetic gases may lead to abortion or fetal mal-formation, the evidence for this is inconclusive. During the first half of

Table 30.1 Sources of pain relief in labour.

Education
    Antenatal classes
        Information
        Demonstrations

Environment
    Pleasant surroundings
    Supportive helpful staff
    Support of partner

Physical methods
    Massage
    Acupuncture
    Transcutaneous electrical nerve stimulation (TENS)

Pharmacological
    Analgesia
        Inhalational, e.g. nitrous oxide
        Narcotic, e.g. pethidine
        Regional analgesia: epidural, spinal, pudendal, perineal infiltration

pregnancy intra-abdominal surgery increases the risk of abortion, but this is probably due to uterine manipulation rather than the anaesthetic agents.

PAIN RELIEF IN LABOUR

The important aspects of pain relief in labour are outlined in Table 30.1.

Although in this chapter interventional management is emphasized, the most important aspect of pain relief in labour is each individual woman's attitude. The ideal approach is for women to be healthy, relaxed, supported by labour partners, fully acquainted with the choice of methods available, free to make a choice, and with open minds should circumstances alter. It is the role of antenatal education to provide women with the opportunity to achieve such a state at the onset of labour.

Physical methods

The major advantage of these methods is that they are non-invasive and therefore not harmful to the fetus. They are useful early in labour and probably act by overloading sensory inputs. Their major disadvantage is that they are often ineffective later in labour.

Inhalational agents

Entonox (50% nitrous oxide, 50% oxygen) is the only inhalational agent now available. The advantages of these agents are that they are self-administered and of almost no danger to mother or fetus. The major disadvantage is that they are commonly used incorrectly leading to failure of this method.

In active labour, although contractions last approximately 60 seconds, the first 20–30 seconds are not usually as painful. It takes a similar period of time, 20–30 seconds, of deep panting using Entonox to achieve a blood level sufficient for analgesia. It is therefore important for the woman to begin rapid respiration with the onset of each contraction rather than waiting until the contraction is painful. Similarly, in the second stage of labour when pain is present throughout contractions, contractions must be anticipated by 30 seconds and inhalation commenced if this method is to be successful.

Narcotic agents

Pethidine is the preferred narcotic for use in labour as it is less soporific than the other narcotics. Although it is a strong analgesic and is easily administered, there is a high incidence of side-effects and 40% of women in labour report no relief of pain. The side-effects are:

1. Dizziness

2. Drowsiness
3. Dissociated state of consciousness
4. Nausea
5. Vomiting
6. Hypotension.

Pethidine is usually given as a bolus i.m. injection of 100 mg which may need to be repeated. It is rare for a woman in labour to require more than two doses and, if the need arises, progress in labour should be reviewed. It is unlikely to cause significant delay in the active phase of labour. The effect on the fetus is to depress heart rate variability and breathing movements and it causes respiratory depression and hypotonicity in the newborn. Respiratory depression is most likely to occur if a narcotic is given i.m. $2\frac{1}{2}$–$3\frac{1}{2}$ hours prior to delivery. Respiratory depression is unlikely more than six hours after i.m. administration. Respiratory depression within six hours of narcotic administration is treated with a narcotic antagonist, most commonly naloxone 20 μg i.m., repeated if necessary. *200 μg IM.*

Because nausea and vomiting are common side-effects of narcotic administration, they are often given with an antiemetic. The antiemetic chosen varies considerably but is either an antihistamine, e.g. promethazine hydrochloride, an antidopaminergic (phenothiazine), e.g. prochlorperazine, or metoclopramide. The first two have sedative and anxiolytic properties and are sometimes preferred because of these effects.

The routine use of other sedatives, e.g. diazepam or barbiturates is not acceptable in modern obstetric practice because of their prolonged effect on the neonate.

Epidural analgesia

The epidural (or extradural) space is the potential space lying outside the dura mater and containing blood vessels, lymphatics and fat. The injection of local anaesthetics into this space produces analgesia in the spinal nerve roots to which the anaesthetic agents diffuse. Therefore, to provide effective analgesia in the first stage of labour the T10–L1 nerve roots must be blocked, while in the second stage of labour the sacral roots must be blocked. The use of epidural analgesia for caesarean section requires a more extensive block to at least T8 and sometimes even T6. There are two routes for epidural analgesia: caudal via the sacrococcygeal membrane or lumbar between adjacent vertebral spines. In obstetrics the latter route is now used almost exclusively.

Indications

1. Pain relief. This is the commonest reason.
2. Hypertensive disorders. Blood pressure is more easily controlled when an effective epidural block is present.

3. Maternal heart disease. The abolition of pain reduces stress and the bearing down reflex thereby relieving strain on the heart. Care is necessary, however, if the patient has a fixed cardiac output, e.g. mitral or aortic stenosis, and cannot compensate for hypotension.
4. Cerebrovascular disease. This is rare in pregnancy but epidural analgesia would be indicated in the presence of an intracranial aneurysm or angioma.
5. Breech and twin delivery. The presence of an effective epidural block allows the use of forceps to control delivery of the aftercoming head in a breech delivery and intrauterine manipulation of the second twin.

Contraindications

1. Recent antepartum haemorrhage. Epidural analgesia may be associated with profound hypotension in the presence of significant blood loss.
2. Coagulation disorder. Clotting defects due to anticoagulants or coagulopathy (e.g. in severe pre-eclampsia) increase the risk of haemorrhage into the epidural space.
3. Sepsis at the injection site.
4. Sensitivity to local anaesthetic agents.
5. Lack of adequately trained staff.
6. Bony disorder of lower spine.
7. Active neurological disease.

In the presence of a uterine scar (previous caesarean section or hysterotomy) some obstetricians will not offer epidural analgesia. This is because of the concern that the epidural may 'mask' the pain of uterine rupture. This is a subject of debate and in most units epidural analgesia is used in the presence of a uterine scar.

Management

A fine plastic catheter is passed through an introducer which is inserted in the midline midway between two lumbar spinous processes—usually L2–3 or L3–4 (Fig. 30.1). Positioning of the patient is critical and the epidural catheter is inserted when the woman is lying in the left lateral position or, less commonly, sitting with her back flexed. The skin area is cleansed and the large bore Tuohy needle (introducer) is inserted after the skin and subcutaneous tissues are infiltrated with local anaesthetic.

The commonest local anaesthetic agent used is bupivacaine. Bupivacaine is given (5–20 ml of 0.25%, 0.375% or 0.5%) in an initial test dose of 3 ml and then five minutes later the remainder is given. The purpose of giving a test dose is to ensure that the catheter has not inadvertently traversed the dura (a spinal block) or is in an epidural vein. Lignocaine is used less commonly and provides a shorter acting, dense block which is useful prior to instrumental delivery.

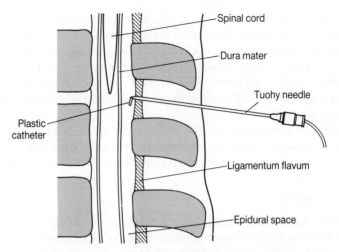

Fig. 30.1   The correct insertion of an epidural catheter. A Tuohy needle is pushed through the skin and ligamentum flavum into the epidural space. The plastic catheter is then passed through the needle, pushed a little further into the space, and the needle is removed.

Observations

Prior to inserting the epidural catheter an i.v. line must be inserted and hypovolaemia corrected. The use of a 'preload' of 500–1000 ml crystalloid fluid is controversial. The fetal heart must be monitored continuously and blood pressure and pulse recorded every five minutes for at least 15 minutes. An analgesic effect is not observed for 15–20 minutes and usually lasts 60–90 minutes. As soon as sensation begins to return the epidural catheter should be 'topped up'. An alternative method is to attach the catheter to a syringe pump and give a continuous infusion of anaesthetic agent.

Complications

1. Hypotension (drop in systolic blood pressure of > 20 mmHg) is treated by ensuring that aortocaval compression is not occurring and administering one litre of Hartmann's solution or normal saline over 20 minutes. If these measures are ineffective or maternal or fetal distress occur, ephedrine should be given, 5–10 mg i.v. This has an inotropic and chronotropic action on the heart and does not cause placental vaso-constriction.
2. Total spinal block occurs with injection of the local anaesthetic agent into the intrathecal space. There is rapid block of motor, sensory and autonomic nerves. This is manifested by marked hypotension, bradycardia and progressive respiratory distress culminating in apnoea. Treatment is to provide oxygen and vasopressors initially and, if complete respiratory paralysis occurs, artificial ventilation.

3. Failure to achieve adequate analgesia can usually be treated by injecting further anaesthetic but if this fails, the epidural catheter may have to be resited.

4. Dural puncture occurs in 1–2% of cases and results in a severe headache in 70% of these cases. The headache usually starts within 48 hours of delivery and lasts for six days if left untreated. If it is recognized at the time of insertion the catheter is resited and good analgesia achieved. The puncture is treated by an infusion of 1.5 l of crystalloid solution into the epidural catheter for 24–36 hours following delivery. An elective forceps delivery should be performed if delivery is not speedily effected. If the saline instillation is ineffective a 'blood patch' is performed. A blood clot over the hole in the dura is achieved by injecting 20 ml of the patient's blood into the epidural space. The patient lies flat for 30 minutes and the headache is usually absent after this period.

5. Increased rate of forceps delivery. There is still considerable debate on this issue. The aggressive use of syntocinon in the second stage of labour will reduce the forceps rate. Despite syntocinon, there appears to be an increased rate of both straight and rotational forceps deliveries with epidurals but this does not increase the perinatal morbidity or mortality.

6. Local anaesthesic toxicity may develop with either accidental intra-vascular injection or excessive total dosage. Premonitory signs include a metallic taste, circumoral tingling, nervousness and nausea. If un-treated, these may progress to muscle twitching leading to convulsions, cardiovascular depression and cardiac arrest.

7. Other rare complications are meningitis and neurological sequelae.

The major advantage of epidural analgesia is that it is the only method of completely abolishing pain in labour (90% of patients have complete or substantial relief). The fetus is rarely affected and the patient is awake and alert. The major disadvantage is that it requires the presence of skilled personnel. Closer observation is also necessary and there is an increased incidence of operative delivery.

Caesarean section. As discussed above, caesarean section under epidural anaesthesia requires a more extensive block. The advantages are that the patient and her partner can see and be involved with the infant immediately; blood loss is reduced and the incidence of postoperative complications is reduced. The disadvantages are that the anaesthesia may not be sufficient necessitating general anaesthesia and, from the operator's point of view, the baby is more difficult to deliver as the patient's abdominal muscles may not be completely relaxed.

Spinal analgesia

Spinal block is used primarily as a single injection intrathecally in the lumbar region for instrumental delivery or caesarean section. A small volume (1.5 ml) of a heavy form of local anaesthetic agent is injected with patient in the sitting position to minimize the spread of the agent cephalically. The block is effective in 3–5 minutes and the patient is observed as with epidural anaesthesia. The advantage of this method is that it is rapid and gives a dense block. The disadvantages are that if it is ineffective then there is no catheter to repeat the dose and cephalic spread with consequent respiratory depression may occur.

Pudendal block

This is a suitable method of analgesia for non-rotational forceps or vacuum extraction. The pudendal nerve is blocked by infiltrating 5–10 ml of 0.5–1% lignocaine around the nerve on each side as it passes around the ischial spine. This is usually done vaginally or, rarely, through the perineum. The commonest problem is that there may be inadequate analgesia on one or both sides and perineal infiltration is often required.

GENERAL ANAESTHESIA

The major problems associated with general anaesthesia in the obstetric patient are regurgitation and aspiration of the stomach contents during induction of anaesthesia. Although this has been recognized for many years it is still a major cause of avoidable maternal death. The reasons for the increased risk are:

1. General anaesthesia is often performed as an emergency procedure with the patient not starved.
2. There is delayed gastric emptying and relaxation of the lower oesophageal sphincter in pregnancy.
3. In labour, gastric emptying is even further delayed especially when opioids are given.
4. Oedema of the vocal cords is more common in pregnancy (due to pre-eclampsia).
5. The increase in body fat and breast size in pregnancy and the presence of an abdominal mass combine to make intubation technically more difficult.

Indications

1. Early pregnancy—abortion, termination of pregnancy, ectopic pregnancy, insertion of cervical suture.
2. Caesarean section.
3. Instrumental delivery—this is rarely necessary under general anaesthesia and should be used with great caution because of the risk of fetal trauma.

4. Obstetric emergencies—ruptured or inverted uterus, uncontrollable postpartum haemorrhage.
5. Manual removal of the placenta.

Preoperative medication

The drugs usually given preoperatively are contraindicated in pregnancy because of the effects on the fetus. Acidity of the stomach contents is reduced by giving H2-receptor blocking drugs orally every six hours in labour and prior to elective surgery in pregnancy. Ranitidine is more commonly used as it has fewer side effects than cimetidine. An alkali mixture, e.g. 15–30 ml magnesium trisilicate or sodium citrate, is given orally immediately prior to induction of anaesthesia.

Induction of anaesthesia

The patient is placed in the left lateral position during transport to, and in, the anaesthetic room. Oxygen is given by mask or mouthpiece for 3–5 minutes prior to induction. This reduces the effects on mother and fetus of the apnoeic period between the onset of paralysis and the initiation of ventilation.

Following the injection of the induction agent, cricoid pressure is immediately applied and maintained until the endotracheal tube is in place and its cuff inflated. The most commonly used induction agent is thiopentone (250–300 mg). This is followed immediately by suxamethonium to induce rapid paralysis to allow endotracheal intubation. Paralysis is continued throughout the operation and anaesthesia maintained with nitrous oxide in oxygen which is administered in a relatively high concentration until delivery has occurred. This mixture is supplemented with a volatile agent in low concentrations.

Following delivery, syntocinon (5–10 mg) is given to ensure uterine contraction.

Complications

Because light anaesthesia is maintained prior to delivery, approximately 3% of patients will experience some degree of awareness of which about one-tenth will be painful. This dilemma is difficult to resolve because of the concern over neonatal drug-induced CNS depression. The use of volatile 0.5% halothane or an equivalent dose of isoflurane or enthrane virtually abolishes awareness.

Aspiration of gastric contents (Mendelson's syndrome) is the most important contributor to maternal morbidity and mortality associated with general anaesthesia. The syndrome is unlikely to occur if the pH of the gastric contents is > 3.0, stressing the importance of prophylactic measures discussed above. Management involves bronchoscopy if solid material is aspirated, oxygen and bronchodilators, intravenous fluids, steroids and antibiotics, and artificial ventilation if necessary.

Other complications of general anaesthesia are:

1. Intraoperative
   a. Circulatory collapse
   b. Respiratory failure
   c. Cardiac failure.
2. Postoperative
   a. Patient drowsy
   b. Respiratory infection
   c. Deep venous thrombosis/pulmonary embolus
   d. Gastrointestinal stasis.

31. Puerperium and breast-feeding

G. Davis

Expectations of the examiners

Problems arising in the puerperium are usually managed in the community and therefore by general practitioners. The examiners will expect candidates to have a good understanding of the normal course of the puerperium and practical remedies for any problems. The management of postpartum haemorrhage is a frequent examination question as it is a life-threatening condition which is relatively common.

Definitions

Puerperium: the weeks following delivery in which the pregnancy-induced changes return to normal. By convention this is six weeks although it may take longer for all the organs to return to normal.

Postpartum haemorrhage (PPH).

Primary: blood loss from the genital tract of 500 ml or more in the first 24 hours after delivery.

Secondary: blood loss from the genital tract of 500 ml or more at any time in the puerperium after the first 24 hours.

Puerperal pyrexia: temperature of 38°C or greater, or 37.4°C on three successive days, within 14 days of delivery or miscarriage.

Physiology

The pelvic organs never entirely return to normal after childbirth. The uterus weighs 1000–1200 g immediately postpartum, 500 g one week later, and has returned to the non-pregnant weight (50–70 g) by six weeks. It is not normally palpable abdominally after 10–14 days. The cervix never returns to normal and is slit-like and often irregular. Mature breast milk is produced by seven days postpartum as a result of oestrogen withdrawal.

The increased production of plasma proteins which occurs in pregnancy rapidly returns to normal after delivery and this is complete by three weeks postpartum. The cardiovascular and renal systems have returned to their non-pregnant state by six weeks, except the renal collecting system which takes about three months. The cardiovascular system reverts quickly after delivery and is 50% back to normal by the third day after delivery.

Ovulation after delivery is extremely variable and affected by lactation. In non-lactating women, 10–15% will have ovulated by 6 weeks and 30% by 13 weeks. In lactating women, ovulation is rare before 10 weeks. Menstruation often occurs prior to initial ovulation.

POSTPARTUM HAEMORRHAGE

PRIMARY

See Labour—Third stage (Ch. 25).

SECONDARY

Secondary PPH is not usually as life-threatening as primary PPH but can be very frightening to the patient.

Aetiology

1. Infection
2. Retained products of conception.

Assessment

1. History
   a. Amount of blood loss—as most cases occur at home this is often difficult to assess
   b. Method of delivery
   c. Completeness of placenta at delivery
   d. Fever
   e. Offensive lochia
2. Examination
   a. Temperature, other vital signs
   b. Height and tenderness of fundus
   c. State of the cervical os
3. Investigations
   a. USS will sometimes demonstrate retained products of conception but is usually not helpful in those cases where it is not clinically obvious.
   b. FBC, cross-match
   c. Cervical swabs
   d. Blood cultures and other investigations as required if the patient is septicaemic.

Treatment

In most cases the diagnosis is clear—if the cervical os is open then evacuation of the uterus will be necessary. If the woman is febrile and/or toxic then 12–24 hours of intravenous antibiotics are required prior to the evacuation. A tender well retracted uterus with a closed cervical os in an otherwise well woman should be treated with oral antibiotics, amoxycillin and metronidazole (200 mg t.d.s. in breast-feeding women).

PUERPERAL INFECTION

Interesting facts

This was the largest cause of maternal mortality until the 1930s when aseptic techniques, and then antibiotics were introduced. Puerperal fever was caused by the spread of group A streptococcus from patient to patient. Anaemia increases the susceptibility of women to infection postnatally.

Pathophysiology

Although infection may occur at any site, the puerperal woman is particularly susceptible to wound infection and infection of the reproductive, urinary and respiratory tracts and the breasts.

1. The reproductive tract has usually been traumatized and there may be retained products or blood clot. In practice, the severity of infection is varied:
   a. Mild infection confined to the vagina, cervix and uterus
   b. Moderate infection with spread to the pelvic organs to give salpingitis and pelvic peritonitis
   c. Severe cases where generalized peritonitis and septicaemia develop.
2. The urinary collecting system is still dilated and the woman may have been catheterized during delivery.
3. General anaesthesia predisposes the woman to postnatal chest infection.
4. The breasts become engorged after delivery and bacterial contamination and infection may occur.
5. The presence of an abdominal wound after caesarean section is a focus for infection.

Bacteriology

1. Reproductive tract
   a. Endogenous organisms
      i. Coliforms
      ii. *Streptococcus faecalis*

    iii. Anaerobic streptococci
    iv. *Clostridium welchii*
  b. Exogenous organisms
    i. Haemolytic streptococcus (group A)
    ii. *Staphylococcus aureus*
2. Urinary tract
  a. *Escherichia coli* (90%)
  b. Others
    i. *Proteus*
    ii. *Klebsiella*
3. Breasts
  a. *Staphylococcus aureus* (> 90%).

Assessment

Women with puerperal pyrexia need a full history, physical examination, diagnosis of the source of infection and appropriate treatment.

History

1. Method of delivery
2. History of trauma to birth canal
3. Time of onset of fever (infections in the birth canal usually give a rise in temperature 12–24 hours after delivery)
4. Site of pain
5. Any other symptoms suggesting incidental infection, e.g. sore throat.

Examination

A full physical examination should be made with particular attention to:

1. Signs of septicaemia
  a. Temperature
  b. Rapid, weak pulse
  c. Hypotension
  d. Pallor
  e. Altered consciousness.
2. Chest—signs of infection
3. Abdomen
  a. The fundus may be tender and high if endometritis is present
  b. More widespread tenderness *or* peritonism is associated with severe puerperal sepsis
  c. The abdominal wound is the commonest site of infection after caesarean section
4. Vagina
  a. The perineum should be inspected

b. If the cervical os is dilated then retained products are likely.
5. Lower limbs
   Deep venous thrombosis (DVT) is more common in the postnatal period and may cause pyrexia. The pelvic veins may be involved, particularly if sepsis is present.

Investigations

1. Midstream specimen of urine
2. High vaginal/endocervical swabs for culture
3. Blood cultures if temperature $> 38°C$
4. Other investigations if septicaemic
5. Venogram (or USS if available) if suspicion of DVT
6. Sputum if chest infection is suspected
7. Wound swab if abdominal delivery.

Treatment

1. Reproductive tract. Evacuation of retained products should be performed after 12–24 hours of i.v. antibiotics. Septicaemia will need appropriate circulatory support and often these patients are best managed in an intensive care unit. Treatment should begin before the infecting agent or its sensitivities are known, but after appropriate swabs have been taken.
   a. Mild
      i. Amoxycillin (oral)
      ii. Metronidazole (oral)
   b. Moderate
      i. Ampicillin (i.v.)
      ii. Metronidazole (pr)
   c. Severe
      i. Cefuroxime (i.v.)
      ii. Gentamicin (i.v.)
      iii. Metronidazole (pr).
2. Urinary tract
   a. Amoxycillin, or
   b. Nitrofurantoin—this is more effective than amoxycillin but there is a small risk of haemolysis in patients with G6PD deficiency
   c. Pyelonephritis requires i.v. cefuroxime or ampicillin.
3. Breast infection. See Breast-feeding.
4. Chest infection
   a. Amoxycillin, or
   b. Erythromycin
   c. Other antibiotics as appropriate.

OTHER PROBLEMS

Thrombosis

There is an increased risk of thrombosis in the puerperium because of the hypercoaguable state of the blood (oestrogen effect) and other predisposing factors: pelvic trauma during delivery, bed rest, varicose veins. If there is any suspicion of DVT or pulmonary embolus, full heparin anticoagulation is indicated and urgent definitive investigation. Warfarin passes into breast milk but in such small quantities that breast-feeding is not contraindicated.

Haemorrhoids

The venodilatation that occurs in pregnancy is exacerbated by the woman's expulsive efforts in labour and haemorrhoids are a common problem in the first few days postpartum. The treatment is conservative with the use of salt baths and proprietary soothing agents. Advice on a high fibre and fluid diet should be given. Prolapsed haemorrhoids should be replaced after each bowel movement. Surgery, except in extreme cases, should only be performed when the problem still persists three months after delivery.

Psychiatric complications

The 'blues' begin on day 2–3 after delivery in 50% of women. Clinical depression occurs in 5% and frank puerperal psychosis in 0.3%. The cause of these disturbances is unknown but the high incidence suggests a metabolic cause. Risk factors are:

1. Previous postpartum psychiatric disorder
2. Previous psychiatric history
3. Previous stillbirth or early neonatal death
4. Ambivalence about motherhood or relationship with her partner
5. Lack of social contacts
6. Major problem in the pregnancy or puerperium.

Features of the blues are lability of mood, anxiety, tiredness and insomnia. They are best treated by education, support and night sedation if sleeping is a problem. Any sign of more severe psychiatric disturbance should precipitate early referral to psychiatric services. Depression may become evident at any time up to 3–4 months postnatally and is recognized by tiredness, insomnia, psychomotor slowing, loss of confidence and a withdrawal from relationships with partner and/or baby. Treatment involves restructuring the woman's daily life so that she has adequate rest, and counselling and specialist referral may be required.

Psychosis is rare, usually depressive in nature and can be life-threatening to mother, baby or both. Urgent psychiatric referral and care is required and the best results are achieved if mother and baby remain together.

BREAST-FEEDING

Physiology

The principal hormone involved in milk biosynthesis is prolactin but complete development of the terminal alveolar cells of the breast into active milk-secreting units also requires insulin, cortisol, oestrogen and progesterone. During pregnancy, prolactin, which is secreted by the anterior pituitary, increases from eight weeks to reach its maximum at term. Human placental lactogen (HPL) is secreted by the placenta in huge amounts and may have some lactogenic effect but its major role in pregnancy is in the regulation of lipolysis. Full lactation in pregnancy is prevented by high levels of progesterone which interfere with the binding of prolactin to its receptors in the glandular tissue of the breast.

During pregnancy, and for the first 3–4 days after delivery, only colostrum is produced, consisting of desquamated, epithelial cells and a transudate from maternal serum. The trigger for full milk secretion is the rapid clearance of oestrogen and progesterone which occurs after delivery. Prolactin levels also fall but more slowly. Suckling initiates milk 'let-down' by stimulating tactile sensors in the areolae which cause oxytocin release from the posterior pituitary. The blood-borne oxytocin causes the myoepithelial cells in the breast ductal system to contract and eject stored milk. Suckling also stimulates prolactin secretion which is necessary for the on-going synthesis of milk. Optimal milk production depends on the availability of thyroxine, insulin, cortisol, dietary intake of nutrients and fluid, frequent feeding and a supportive environment. As a general principle, 1% of any drug administered to the mother will cross to the infant.

Composition

Colostrum is a yellow fluid with a high content of antibodies, particularly secretory IgA. It contains more protein (desquamated cells) but less carbohydrate and fat than normal breast milk. Most of the protein is lactalbumin and casein with the lactalbumin providing the essential amino acids (Table 31.1).

In extreme circumstances, the high levels of sodium and phosphorus in cow's milk may lead, respectively, to hypernatraemia in infants with diarrhoea, and low calcium and convulsions. Preterm babies need larger amounts of sodium, calcium and phosphorus.

Management

Antenatal

Patients should be encouraged to breast-feed, and general health and diet should be maintained. Nipple shields may be of some value to women with

Table 31.1   Composition of milk. (From T E Oppe 1974 Present day practice of infant feeding. DHSS Report on Health and Social Subjects. London, HMSO.)

	Human	Cow
Protein	1.0 g/dl	3.3 g/dl
Fat	3.8 g/dl	3.7 g/dl
Carbohydrate	7 g/dl	4.8 g/dl
Sodium	15 mg/dl	58 mg/dl
Calcium	33 mg/dl	125 mg/dl
Phosphorus	15 mg/dl	96 mg/dl
Energy	67 kcal/dl	66 kcal/dl

inverted nipples. Daily antenatal care of the nipples is probably not of great benefit.

Postpartum

The mother and infant should have learned how to breast-feed by 3–4 days postpartum when normal milk production begins. It can be a stressful time for both partners so gentle reassurance, supervision and education by an experienced person is optimal. Mother and infant should be comfortable and the mother should have washed her hands. The nipple (including part of the areola) is fed into the baby's mouth and the nose is kept clear by the mother pressing a finger on the breast just above the baby's nose. The 'let-down reflex' occurs in the first three minutes and the infant obtains 90% of its feed in the first 3–5 minutes. When the infant is finished, the nipple is gently withdrawn and the baby is 'winded'. Feeding is most effective if the infant is fed when hungry rather than to a schedule.

Problems

Engorgement

This is due to the sudden secretion of milk on the third or fourth day and is best avoided by frequent feeding under supervision. Treatment is to use heat in the form of a shower or bath, analgesia, a firm, supportive brassiere and reassurance. Sometimes expression of a small amount of milk relieves tension in the breast sufficiently for the infant to fix on the nipple adequately.

Infection

Mastitis. This usually occurs as a result of a cracked nipple or a blocked duct. There is a tender, inflamed wedge of breast tissue and a pyrexia. *Staphylococcus aureus* is the cause of 95% of mastitis, and it should be treated with flucloxacillin or erythromycin. Breast-feeding should continue unless this is too painful, in which case milk should be expressed from the affected breast.

Abscess. Abscesses usually develop if mastitis is not treated promptly or correctly. Fluctuance may be difficult to elicit but an abscess should be suspected if mastitis does not resolve with antibiotics. The treatment of the abscess is to stop breast-feeding from the infected side, continue expressing the milk and incision and drainage.

Nipples

Problems with nipples are one of the major reasons for women giving up breast-feeding and therefore should be treated assiduously.

Pain. Pain is experienced by 80% of women 2–4 days after delivery. This is usually associated with engorgement and is treated by more frequent, brief feeds, keeping the nipples clean and exposing the nipple to air (breast shields) and to sunlight.

Cracked nipples. Superficial cracks are treated as above but with deep cracks, the baby should be temporarily removed and the breast gently expressed by hand until it heals. Antiseptic sprays or creams are not useful.

Contraception

If breast-feeding is used exclusively and menstruation does not appear, ovulation usually does not occur before the eleventh week postpartum. Menstruation resumes in 40–75% of women while still breast-feeding and ovulation occurs shortly after. The contraceptive effectiveness of lactation depends on the frequency of suckling, the use of supplemental feeding and the level of maternal nutrition (if low, the contraceptive effectiveness is greater). As oestrogens inhibit prolactin release their use in the postpartum period is contraindicated although many women will continue to breast-feed normally if commenced on the combined oral contraceptive once breast-feeding is well established.

The other options for contraception are: progestogens (the progestogen only pill (POP) or Depo-Provera), barrier methods, or IUCDs. Most women opt for the POP which should be started in the first postpartum week. Its commonest complications are irregular bleeding and a higher failure rate compared to the combined pill or Depo-Provera.

Suppression of lactation

In most cases, this is achieved by not stimulating the breasts (no suckling), a firm supportive brassiere and analgesia if required. By 5–6 days postpartum the discomfort improves. Complete suppression of lactation can be achieved with bromocryptine 2.5 mg b.d. for 10–14 days followed by gradual withdrawal over the ensuing seven days. Lactation suppression is indicated in perinatal death, adoption of the infant, severe breast problems, or active maternal tuberculosis. Routine use is not recommended because of the side-effects of nausea and vomiting and reports of hypertension, stroke and myocardial infarction associated with the postpartum use of bromocryptine.

OTHER PUERPERAL CONSIDERATIONS

Contraception

Contraception in breast-feeding women is discussed above. In women who are not breast-feeding, 50% will ovulate prior to the six week postnatal check so contraception should be instituted in the first three weeks after delivery. In the non-lactating woman the choices are similar to that for the non-puerperal woman.

Vaccinations

All women lacking rubella antibodies should be vaccinated after delivery providing contraception can be assured for the ensuing three months. All rhesus-negative women delivering rhesus-positive babies should be given Anti-D prophylaxis (not strictly a vaccination) within 72 hours of delivery.

Postnatal examination

This is traditionally performed at six weeks postpartum as most of the pregnancy-induced changes in maternal physiology have returned to normal and it is an appropriate time for assessing the mother–infant interaction.

As mentioned above, contraception in the non-lactating woman should have been initiated prior to this visit. At the visit a brief history should be taken focusing on the maternal reproductive tract, breasts and the infant's feeding, behaviour and health. Maternal blood pressure should be checked, particularly if this has been a problem in pregnancy, and the breasts and lower genital tract examined. A smear should be performed if necessary.

32. Home deliveries

I. Page

Expectations of the examiners

The candidate will be expected to be aware of the special arrangements needed for home deliveries, and to appreciate under which circumstances women initially suitable for home delivery should be transferred to specialist care. In addition, the candidate should be able to perform a normal delivery, to recognize abnormalities that may occur in labour, and to resuscitate a mother or baby.

Epidemiology

The place of delivery was first recorded nationally in 1927, when 85% of births took place at home. Successive government committees advocated increasing the proportion of hospital deliveries and in 1984, 96% took place in NHS GP/consultant units, 3% in isolated GP units and 1% at home.

The many advantages that have been claimed for hospital delivery are now being reassessed.

Assessment

Every woman has the right to have her baby at home, and health authorities are required to ensure a midwifery service for home births is provided.

The assessment of suitability for a home delivery must cover two aspects: 1. the anticipated 'normality' of the delivery for the mother and baby and 2. the adequacy of facilities in the home.

Home facilities

These are usually assessed by the midwife who will be undertaking the delivery. The birth room must be heated to, and maintained at, about 22°C. It should be clean and well lit. A work-top of some form will be necessary for the midwife's equipment. If the woman intends to give birth on her bed, the mattress must be firm to allow the midwife access to the woman's perineum.

Ideally, a telephone should be present in the house to enable the midwife to summon help immediately if it is required. A neighbour's telephone is acceptable, providing there is easy access to it.

Hot water should be available, as should a means of warming the blankets and clothes the baby will wear (a hot water bottle is adequate).

Obstetric assessment

Broad guidelines regarding the place of delivery were laid down by the Maternity Services (Cranbrook) Committee in 1959 and are still applicable. Their aim is to try to avoid transfer of the mother and baby during labour, as this has been shown to worsen the outcome. Where there is an apparent medical or obstetric contraindication to home delivery, the midwife and GP should encourage the woman to have a consultant's opinion. Ultimately, if the woman decides to have the baby at home, the midwife *must* attend. She can call on *any* GP in an emergency who will be bound to attend, or she can request the assistance of the local obstetric (or paediatric) flying squad (see Appendix 1).

Height. Women under 152 cm (5 ft 0 in) have a higher PNMR, and a higher incidence of caesarean section in labour.

Age. Nulliparae under 18 years or over 30 years are known to have an increased PNMR, as do multiparous women over 35 years.

Parity. Nulliparae are known to have an increased incidence of prolonged labour which makes intrapartum transfer more likely. They are also more likely to develop pre-eclampsia, and to require induction of labour for prolonged pregnancy.

'Grand multiparae' have an increased risk of multiple pregnancy, placenta praevia, fetal malpresentation and unstable lie. There is an increased risk of disproportion, which may present as uterine rupture or shoulder dystocia. Paradoxically, the uterus tends to relax more in the third stage, giving rise to an increased risk of postpartum haemorrhage.

Weight. Obese women are more difficult to assess as 'normal' in pregnancy and labour, and often have large babies. It is more difficult to treat them if problems arise.

Social class. This is becoming harder to assess, but social classes IV and V are at increased risk of maternal, fetal or neonatal problems.

Maternal disease. Any coexisting disease, such as hypertension or diabetes mellitus, is a contraindication to home delivery.

Previous uterine surgery. A scar in the uterus (previous caesarean section, hysterotomy or myomectomy) is at risk of dehiscence which may require urgent major surgery.

Obstetric history. Any woman who has suffered a previous perinatal loss should not be booked for home delivery. Similarly, previous low birth-weight babies (whether due to prematurity or growth retardation) or difficult deliveries are contraindications to home delivery, as are problems in the third stage (PPH, retained placenta) which have an increased risk of recurrence.

Current pregnancy. If the pregnancy becomes abnormal then care should be transferred to the hospital antenatally. Abnormalities can occur at any stage of pregnancy, and examples include isoimmunization, pre-eclampsia, antepartum haemorrhage, malpresentation (after 37 weeks), multiple pregnancy and fetal growth retardation.

Summary

A healthy woman, over 152 cm tall, under 35 years of age, having had a previously normal pregnancy and delivery, having her second to fourth baby, in social class I, II or III and with no current medical or obstetric problems can be defined as 'low-risk' and home delivery viewed as acceptable.

Advantages

Many of the claimed advantages for home delivery are difficult, if not impossible, to quantify as they refer to the way the mother feels about the birth. It is certainly true to say that being treated as an individual is more likely at home, as most hospitals have policies of management which have been designed to cope with the abnormal and do not need to be applied to low-risk cases.

Disadvantages

The incidence of serious, unexpected emergencies that can harm the mother and her baby is about 7%, even in low-risk cases. They include fetal distress, shoulder dystocia, neonatal apnoea, postpartum haemorrhage and retained placenta. Some of them can, however, be managed adequately by the attending midwife.

The major problems arise in those cases where urgent medical assistance and skill is required. In these cases there may be some considerable delay awaiting the arrival of the GP or local flying squad, during which time the condition of the mother or baby may markedly deteriorate.

SUMMARY

Home delivery is now a rare event. It can be accepted for 'low-risk' mothers providing the attending midwife makes adequate arrangements for assistance in an emergency. In addition, the woman and her partner should have a full understanding of the risks and benefits of a home delivery.

33. Maternity benefits

I. Page

Expectations of the examiners

The candidate will be expected to be aware of the various benefits which are available to pregnant women and mothers.

Accuracy

Details of the benefits change with the Chancellor's budget each year. The details below follow the 1989 Budget.

DURING PREGNANCY

Dental treatment

Details are set out in leaflet D11—NHS dental treatment. Free dental treatment is available during pregnancy and for 12 months after delivery. It is also available for anyone receiving family credit or income support (see below). Form F1D, available from the dental surgery, should be completed even if the woman is receiving either family credit or income support to ensure she can receive free treatment for the full period if she should stop being eligible for the benefit.

Prescription charges

Details are set out in leaflet P11—NHS prescriptions. A prescription charge exemption certificate is available during pregnancy and for 12 months afterwards. Form FW8, which is available from GP surgeries or midwives, should be completed even if the woman is receiving family credit or income support (as with dental treatment).

Hospital fares

Although not strictly a maternity benefit, women receiving family credit or income support can claim public transport fares, petrol costs or occasionally taxi fares for their antenatal (and postnatal) visits. Details are set out in leaflet H11—NHS hospital travel costs. The claim is paid at the hospital on production of the benefit order book. If the woman has a low income she can apply to the agency benefits unit of the DHSS (using form AG1—Help with NHS costs) which may issue a certificate of entitlement.

Social fund maternity payment

Details are set out in leaflets FB8—Babies and benefits, and FB27—Bringing up children? It is intended to help with expenses for the new baby, and can only be made to women receiving family credit or income support. The amount is £85.00 for each baby expected, adopted or born but is reduced if the claimant or her partner hold over £500 in savings. Form SF100, available from antenatal clinics or Social Security offices, should be completed between 11 weeks before and 13 weeks after delivery.

Statutory maternity pay (SMP)

Details are set out in leaflets FB8—Babies and benefits, and NI17A—A guide to maternity benefits. Maternity pay is paid by the woman's employer.

To qualify, the woman must work for her employer for the 26 weeks up to the 15th week before her estimated date of delivery (EDD) and work one day of that week, and also earn enough during the last 8 weeks to pay class 1 national insurance (NI) contributions.

If she is dismissed before the 15th week before her EDD because of problems in the pregnancy or premature delivery she may still be eligible for SMP.

SMP is paid for up to 18 weeks, starting between 11 and 6 weeks before her EDD. It is not paid while the woman is working so she should be advised to stop working by the 34th week of pregnancy otherwise she will lose some of the benefit.

To claim SMP the woman must:

1. Inform her employer in writing at least 3 weeks before stopping work, that she intends to stop work because of pregnancy and intends to claim SMP.
2. Send her maternity certificate (form Mat B1 available from her midwife or doctor after 26 weeks of pregnancy) to her employer before the end of the third week in which she claims SMP.

SMP is paid at two rates. To qualify for the higher rate (6 weeks at 90% of earnings, then 12 weeks at the standard rate) a woman must have worked more than 2 years full-time or 5 years part-time. The standard rate is paid for the whole 18 weeks to women who have worked between 6 months and 2 years, and is £36.25 per week. Income tax and NI contributions may have to be paid on SMP.

State maternity allowance (SMA)

Details are set out in leaflets FB8—Babies and benefits, and NI17A—A guide to maternity benefits. This allowance is paid by the DHSS.

It is payable to women who have recently changed or given up their jobs, or have recently been self-employed.

To qualify a woman must have paid class 1 or 2 NI contributions for at least 26 of the 52 weeks ending in the 15th week before her EDD. As with SMP it is not paid if the woman is working.

To claim SMA, the woman must complete Form MA1, available from her antenatal clinic or Social Security office, and send it with her form Mat B1 to the Social Security office.

SMA is paid at a standard rate of £33.20 per week.

STILLBIRTHS

If the baby is stillborn (by definition after the 28th week of pregnancy) entitlement to the following benefits is not affected:

1. Free NHS dental treatment
2. Free NHS prescriptions
3. Social fund maternity payment
4. Statutory maternity pay
5. State maternity allowance.

AFTER DELIVERY

Child benefit

Details are set out in leaflets CH1—Child benefit, and CH7—Child benefit for children aged 16 and over. It is payable for every child under 16 (19 if in full-time education) living with the claimant.

Payment is usually by a book of orders which can be cashed at the Post Office every 4 weeks.

The claim form is available from Social Security offices and should be accompanied by the child's birth certificate.

Child benefit is at the time of writing £7.25 per week per child.

One parent benefit

Details are set out in leaflets CH11—One parent benefit, and FB27—Bringing up children? It is an extra benefit which is only payable for one child (usually the first).

Payment is usually by a book of orders which can be cashed at the Post Office every 4 weeks.

The claim form is in leaflet CH11, and the benefit is £5.20 per week.

Widow's mother's allowance

Details are set out in leaflet NP45—A guide to widow's benefits. It can be paid from the time of the husband's death for children for whom the woman receives child benefit, or from the time of delivery if she is widowed while pregnant.

If it is paid, then one parent benefit cannot be claimed.

The claim form (form BW1) is available from Social Security offices, and the allowance is £43.60 per week with an extra £8.95 per week per child.

OTHER BENEFITS

As family credit and income support have been mentioned in relation to most of the benefits payable during pregnancy, they are briefly described here. They are general, not maternity, benefits.

Family credit

Details are set out in leaflet FB27—Bringing up children?, and the claim form FC1—family credit is available from Post and Social Security offices.

It is a tax-free benefit for anyone bringing up one child (or more) and working at least 24 hours per week. The amount varies with income, and is usually payable if the net income is less than £96.50 per week with an extra allowance for each child. It is reduced by savings or capital over £3000. Once the rate has been assessed it remains constant for 26 weeks, regardless of changes in circumstances.

If family credit is paid the family are automatically entitled to:

1. Free NHS dental treatment
2. Vouchers for spectacles
3. Free NHS prescriptions
4. Refund of hospital fares
5. Social fund maternity payment.

Income support

Details are set out in leaflets FB27—Bringing up children?, and SB20—A guide to income support. The claim form SB1—Income support—cash help is available from Post and Social Security offices.

It is a taxable benefit for people who do not have enough money on which to live, and who work less than 24 hours per week. The amount varies with individual circumstances, and is reduced if the claimants have capital or savings over £3000.

If income support is paid, the family are automatically entitled to the same benefits as those on family credit (see above).

34. Statistics

I. Page

Expectations of the examiners

The candidate will be expected to have an understanding of the epidemiology of perinatal and maternal morbidity and mortality as well as ethnic variations, and to understand the importance of accurate obstetric records in clinical audit.

BIRTH RATE

Definition

Total live and stillbirths per year per thousand women aged 15–44 years.

Interesting facts

The birth rate is currently (1989) about 60 in the UK, and is showing a downward trend. This is mainly affected by the 'economy'. All births are registered by a midwife (or doctor) with the area health authority within 36 hours, and the parents must notify the local registrar of births and deaths within 42 days of the birth.

ABORTION

This comprises spontaneous abortions (usually referred to as miscarriages) and induced (legal) abortions.

Definition

Termination of a pregnancy before 28 weeks' gestation with the expulsion of a dead fetus.

Interesting facts

The miscarriage rate is estimated to be about 15% of conceptions. The induced abortion rate is currently about 15 per year per thousand women aged 15–44 years in England and Wales. Induced abortion may only be performed on premises approved by the Secretary of State under the 1967 Abortion Act. Less than 50% of induced abortions are carried out by the NHS. Over 80% of induced abortions are now performed within the first trimester of pregnancy.

STILLBIRTH RATE

5·3/1000

Definition

24.

Number of infants born with no signs of life after 28 weeks' gestation per thousand total births.

Interesting facts

The stillbirth rate is currently (1989) about five in the UK, and is showing a downward trend.

NEONATAL DEATH RATE

3·9/1000 live

Definition

28.

Number of deaths, within 28 days of birth, of all live-born infants (regardless of gestation) per thousand live births.

PERINATAL MORTALITY RATE (PNMR)

Definition

7·6/1000 births.

Number of stillbirths and first-week neonatal deaths per thousand total births.

Interesting facts

The PNMR has been recorded since 1930 in the UK and is currently about 10. It is showing a downward trend, with an acceleration in the rate of improvement.

Epidemiology

Age

PNMR is lowest in the age group 20–24 years. The higher rate in the under 20s reflects the greater number of primigravidae and unmarried mothers and poor acceptance of antenatal care. The increase in PNMR with maternal age reflects the greater incidence of maternal disease (such as diabetes and hypertension) and increased parity.

Parity

A similar 'j-shaped' curve is seen when comparing PNMR with parity, with the lowest PNMR occurring in women in their second pregnancy.

Race

Asians (Indians and Pakistanis) have an increased PNMR reflecting a higher incidence of congenital abnormalities and a mean birth-weight 300 g lower than that of Caucasians.

Black people (Africans and Caribbeans) have an increased PNMR due to sickle cell disease, a higher incidence of pre-eclampsia and eclampsia, a higher rate of twin births, lower social class and a mean birth-weight 120 g lower than that of Caucasians.

Social class

PNMR increases between social classes I and V, with a further increase in unsupported women.

Multiple pregnancy

This predisposes to preterm delivery, pre-eclampsia and low birth-weight and so has an increased PNMR. The problems become greater with each extra fetus.

Aetiology

There are three major determinants of perinatal mortality:

1. Congenital abnormalities
2. Low birth-weight
3. Asphyxia.

However it is more useful to look at the causes as below.

Congenital abnormality

This group accounts for 20% of perinatal deaths in the UK, and most of these are of the central nervous system. These can be detected in the second trimester by measurement of maternal serum alpha-fetoprotein, ultrasound examination of the fetus and amniocentesis where necessary. Other genetic and chromosomal abnormalities can be detected by chorion villus sampling or amniocentesis. Termination of affected pregnancies (where the mother wishes) can be performed.

Isoimmunization

Perinatal deaths from haemolytic disease are now rare. The introduction of routine screening of maternal blood for antibodies (in particular anti-D, anti-c, anti-Kell and anti-Duffy) with follow-up by amniocentesis and assessment of the liquor bilirubin level, or by cordocentesis and fetal blood sampling, allows appropriate treatment to be given.

Pre-eclampsia

This excludes essential and renal hypertension which are usually considered a maternal disease, although both increase the risk of developing superimposed pre-eclampsia. Investigations are aimed at detecting fetal asphyxia and growth retardation, as well as ensuring maternal well-being.

Antepartum haemorrhage

Placenta praevia has little effect on PNMR as few babies require early delivery because of it, and those who are delivered early are usually in good condition.

Abruption is more common and accounts for about 20% of perinatal deaths due to asphyxia and prematurity. The risk of abruption increases with smoking and rising parity. It is associated with hypertension and raised maternal alpha-fetoprotein.

Mechanical

These perinatal deaths may be due to uterine rupture and cord accidents (which usually cause asphyxia) or birth trauma (as in breech delivery, forceps delivery or shoulder dystocia).

Maternal disease

Diabetes mellitus is the maternal condition that causes most perinatal deaths. Others of importance are chronic renal disease, SLE or the presence of the lupus anticoagulant alone, and renal transplantation.

Miscellaneous

These are specific causes which cannot be ascribed to prematurity or asphyxia. Examples include the twin–twin transfusion syndrome, milk inhalation and infections.

Unexplained

These are probably due to asphyxia, for which there may or may not be any evidence. Examples include unexplained intrauterine deaths, deaths from unexplained preterm delivery (including respiratory distress syndrome and intraventricular haemorrhage) and are categorized as being:

1. Term or preterm
2. Normal or small for gestational age.

Unclassifiable

A small group.

Prevention

One of the aims of antenatal care is to detect abnormalities early enough during the pregnancy to allow intervention to improve the likely outcome. This is relatively simple for congenital abnormalities where a careful history coupled with specific investigations, or general screening procedures for the whole population, can identify the abnormal fetus and so allow termination of the pregnancy where desired. It is not possible to cure most abnormalities at present, a situation that is unlikely to change for many years.

Isoimmunization with anti-D should be preventable with rhesus prophylaxis in all pregnant women at risk of sensitization. Care with blood transfusion will reduce the numbers who develop other antibodies.

There is no preventive measure against pre-eclampsia at present, although studies into the use of low-dose aspirin are under way. Early diagnosis and awareness of the risk to the fetus are essential. Treatment of the hypertension is of no benefit to the fetus apart from allowing continuation of the pregnancy until the fetus is mature. Cigarette smoking makes the disease less common, but more severe when it does occur, and also increases the incidence of abruption ending in fetal death.

Fatal trauma to the fetus during delivery should be an avoidable event with correct intrapartum care, as should fatal cord accidents. There is no way of preventing antepartum cord accidents.

Ideally, maternal disorders should have been thoroughly assessed and controlled prior to the pregnancy. This is particularly the case with diabetes mellitus, where poor control increases the risk of congenital abnormality as well as increasing the risk of obstetric complications and sudden intrauterine death.

Provision of appropriate neonatal care facilities was emphasized by both the Sheldon Report (1971) and the Short Reports (1980 and 1985). For the high-risk pregnancy, arrangements should be made for delivery in a major obstetric unit with both special and intensive neonatal care units. If appropriate facilities are not available locally, then in utero transfer is safer for the baby.

Improvement of social and environmental conditions is probably the most important factor in reducing the PNMR, as these are closely linked to both congenital abnormalities and low birth-weight babies.

SUMMARY

Perinatal mortality has fallen for a number of reasons and will fall further with improving socioeconomic conditions. Lack of appropriate care is apparent in up to one-third of perinatal deaths and therefore higher standards of obstetric care should result in a further reduction in PNMR. The special problems of the immigrant population must be remembered, and require further investigation.

MATERNAL MORTALITY RATE

Definition

Number of deaths of women while pregnant, or within 42 days of abortion or delivery, per hundred thousand births.

Interesting facts

In England and Wales all maternal deaths are investigated by senior obstetricians, anaesthetists and pathologists and their findings are presented in the Confidential Enquiry into Maternal Deaths which is published triennially. This enquiry has operated since 1952, and details the causes of death and whether care in each case could be said to be substandard. From 1985 onwards the report will include maternal deaths in Scotland and Northern Ireland.

The rate in the latest report (1982–1984) is 8.6, and has halved every 10 years since the report began. Maternal deaths now comprise only 0.7% of deaths of females aged 15–44 years (in 1952 the figure was 3.9%).

Substandard care

This usually implies one of the following:

1. Failure to recognize predisposing factors
2. Failure to institute prophylactic measures
3. Deficiencies in routine antenatal care
4. Failure to recognize dangerous symptoms or signs
5. Delay in instituting proper management
6. Patient self-neglect.

Classification

The report divides the deaths into three groups:

1. Direct. Death due to an obstetric complication arising during pregnancy, labour or the postpartum period, e.g. amniotic fluid embolism.
2. Indirect. Death due to a pre-existing disease which was made worse by the pregnancy, e.g. maternal cardiac disease.
3. Fortuitous. Death due to factors unrelated to, and not influenced by, the pregnancy, e.g. road traffic accident.

Demographic features

Age

Direct maternal mortality between 1976 and 1984 was lowest in women aged 20–24 years. There was a marked increase in the rate in women aged over 35 years.

Parity

Direct mortality is lowest in women having their second baby, and rises with increasing parity.

Race

Maternal mortality in Britain is commoner in women born outside the UK, particularly if they come from Bangladesh, India or Africa. This is similar to PNMR.

Social class

As this is getting harder to assess accurately, it is no longer included in the report. Previously the mortality rate had been lower in the upper social classes. Failure to attend for antenatal care contributes to some of the difference.

UK Area

There are wide variations in the mortality rate in different areas of the UK, but they have no correlation with the variations in PNMR.

Direct deaths

These account for 57% of the total, and their relative frequencies are shown in Table 34.1.

Table 34.1 Causes of direct deaths in England and Wales, 1982–1984.

Cause	% of deaths
Hypertensive diseases	18
Pulmonary embolism	18
Anaesthesia	14
Amniotic fluid embolism	10
Abortion	8
Ectopic pregnancy	7
Haemorrhage	7
Uterine rupture	2
Genital sepsis	1
Miscellaneous	15

Hypertensive diseases

These were commonest in the first pregnancy and in older women. The cause of death is usually cerebral haemorrhage, oedema or infarction. Care was considered to be substandard in nearly three-quarters of the cases, with failure to control the blood pressure adequately and to deliver the patient expeditiously being the main points.

Pulmonary embolism

One-third of these deaths occurred during the pregnancy and two-thirds afterwards. Caesarean section increases the risk of fatal pulmonary embolism 26-fold compared with vaginal delivery. The risk is also increased by obesity, immobilization, previous thromboembolism and increasing parity. It is markedly higher in women aged over 35 years. There has been little change in the rate over the past 10 years.

Anaesthesia

The number of anaesthetic deaths has decreased markedly, but their percentage contribution to maternal mortality has increased due to the increase in the number of obstetric anaesthetics given. In all cases in the last report care was deemed to have been substandard, usually reflecting the inexperience of junior anaesthetists. Half of the deaths were associated with difficulty with intubation, and one-third with aspiration of stomach contents into the lungs (Mendelson's syndrome).

Amniotic fluid embolism

This has a fatal incidence of 7.4 per million maternities. No cases developed symptoms before labour and there were no cases of substandard care. The condition is commoner in women aged over 35 years and with three or more children. The mortality rate has not changed over the past 15 years.

Abortion

Two-thirds of the deaths were associated with legal induced abortion, where haemorrhage was the commonest cause of death and care substandard in half the cases. The other one-third followed spontaneous abortion where sepsis accounted for three-quarters of the deaths. The risk is increased in women aged over 35 years, but is not related to parity.

Ectopic pregnancy

The death rate has fallen despite the marked increase in the incidence of the condition. There was substandard care in one-third of cases, usually failure to perform a vaginal examination. West Indian and Asian women are at increased risk.

Haemorrhage

This had a fatal incidence of 4.8 per million maternities. Half of the cases were antepartum, one-third postpartum and the others due to other obstetric trauma. Care was deemed to be substandard in one-third of the cases. The risk increases with increasing age and parity, but is lowest in the second pregnancy.

Uterine rupture

The rate is decreasing, and there were no cases due to scar dehiscence in the last report. The commonest problem is traumatic rupture associated with the use of oxytocic agents.

Genital sepsis

The rate is decreasing, but was involved in some cases classified under abortion.

Miscellaneous

There were 21 cases in this group in 1982–1984. In eight of them no cause was found, and in the other 13 the cause was a dangerous and rare condition.

Table 34.2 Causes of indirect deaths in England and Wales, 1982–1984.

Cause	% of deaths
CNS disease	32
Cardiac disease	20
Neoplasia	16
CVS disease	12
Septicaemia	4
Respiratory disease	3
Others	13

Indirect deaths

These account for 29% of the total, and their relative frequencies are shown in Table 34.2.

CNS diseases

Half of these deaths were due to intracranial haemorrhage, one-quarter to cerebral arterial thrombosis and one-quarter to status epilepticus in known epileptics.

Cardiac disease

One-third of these deaths was due to congenital, and two-thirds to acquired disease. In the Western world most of the acquired cardiac disease is the result of ischaemic change, while in the developing countries rheumatic heart disease is more prevalent.

The congenital group all had Eisenmenger's syndrome (or a similar anomaly resulting in pulmonary hypertension) and are most at risk during the puerperium or after abortion.

Those with acquired disease are at similar risk throughout the pregnancy and puerperium.

Neoplasia

In most cases it is not certain that pregnancy has any direct effect on prognosis, apart from sometimes delaying treatment.

CVS disease

All the deaths in this group were due to aneurysm rupture, and it has been suggested that there is a relationship between pregnancy and certain degenerative diseases of arteries.

Septicaemia

of the three cases in 1982–1984, two were due to beta-haemolytic streptococci, presenting initially as tonsillitis.

Respiratory disease

In all cases in this group death was due to pneumonia.

Others

Most of these deaths were suicides, where pregnancy was thought to have been part of the underlying reason.

Fortuitous deaths

These account for the remaining 14% of maternal deaths covered by the Triennial Report. They are excluded from the international definition of maternal mortality.

Late deaths

These occur more than 42 days, but less than one year, after a pregnancy or delivery. They are reviewed in the Triennial Report but excluded from the international definition.

Of the 73 late deaths in 1982–1984, six were classified as direct, 17 indirect and 50 as fortuitous.

Caesarean section

Deaths associated with caesarean section are dealt with as a group in the Triennial Report as it is a major, and increasing intervention in obstetric practice.

In 1982–1984 the death rate was 0.37 per thousand operations. Two-thirds were direct, one-quarter indirect and the remainder fortuitous. Care was deemed to have been substandard in half of the direct deaths. Death was 4.5 times more common after an emergency procedure than after an elective one.

Prevention

The following recommendations have been abridged from the 1982–1984 Triennial Report.

Hypertensive disease

Intervention with hypotensive agents should be considered earlier and premature delivery is often required. Signs of impending eclampsia should not be ignored.

Pulmonary embolism

There is a need for earlier detection of deep venous thrombosis. If thrombosis or embolism is strongly suspected then treatment with intravenous heparin should be started immediately.

Anaesthesia

More experienced anaesthetists and assistants should be available in maternity units.

Abortion

Blood must be readily available for all women undergoing abortion, and the danger of concurrent sterilization recognized. Where damage to the genital tract is known (or strongly suspected) to have occurred, the woman should be kept under observation in hospital for at least 24 hours.

Ectopic pregnancy

The diagnosis must be considered in all women aged 15–44 years with abdominal pain, especially if they have a history of subfertility, pelvic inflammatory disease or tubal surgery (includes sterilization).

Haemorrhage

An experienced surgeon should perform caesarean sections for known placenta praevia. All maternity units should have a plan for the management of catastrophic haemorrhage.

Sepsis

Acute tonsillitis or pharyngitis in pregnancy warrants a throat swab—if a Lancefield group A beta-haemolytic streptococcus is isolated, treatment should be with penicillin.

Epilepsy

Blood levels of anticonvulsants should be monitored throughout the pregnancy and puerperium to ensure the correct dose is being prescribed and taken.

Caesarean section

When problems arise a more senior surgeon or anaesthetist should be involved more quickly.

SUMMARY

Maternal mortality is falling due to the better health of the population and improvements in the obstetric care of the mother. As half of the direct deaths showed evidence of substandard care there is still room for improvement. It should be remembered that a vaginal delivery is usually safer for the mother than a caesarean section.

C. Miscellaneous subjects

35. Neonatal medicine

H. Issler

Expectations of the examiners

The candidate should be competent in neonatal resuscitation and be familiar with common neonatal problems and their management.

A paediatrician should be present at the following deliveries:

1. Multiple delivery
2. Meconium stained liquor or fetal distress
3. Infant of a diabetic mother
4. Instrumental deliveries
5. Malpresentation
6. Preterm delivery
7. Caesarean section
8. Haemolytic disease
9. Fetal abnormality
10. Growth retarded fetus.

DELIVERY

Resuscitation

Most hospitals still use the Apgar score to assess the infant's well-being at birth. Originally described by Virginia Apgar in 1953, the score summates five clinical signs—heart rate, respiratory effort, reflex irritability, muscle tone and colour—at one, five and ten minutes. Although its value as an accurate predictor of neonatal outcome is now being questioned it has certainly provided a useful guide for those babies who may require the facilities of a special care baby unit at least for the first 24 hours.

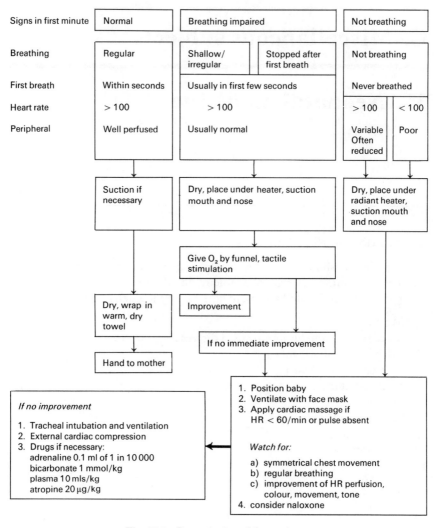

Fig. 35.1 Resuscitation of the newborn.

Routine care

Airway

Should be cleared with a simple sucker.

Temperature control

Heat loss may precipitate respiratory distress. The baby is dried before being wrapped in a warm dry blanket. The head occupies a large surface area and should be covered to prevent heat loss.

Vital statistics

The weight and head circumference are recorded. The umbilical cord is checked for three vessels, two arteries and one vein.

Investigations and treatment

1. Vitamin K 1.0 mg is given orally or by intramuscular injection to prevent haemorrhagic disease of the newborn.
2. Cord blood is taken for blood group, Coombs' test and bilirubin in all infants of rhesus-negative women and where antibodies were detected during the pregnancy.
3. If the mother is known to be hepatitis B positive, particularly E antigen positive with no E antibodies, the baby is passively immunized with antihepatitis B immunoglobulin before leaving the labour ward.

Checklist for newborn

Head

Caput succedaneum, a soft swelling of the scalp, occurs due to compression on the presenting part. This swelling is not related to suture lines and clears spontaneously in a few days.

A cephalhaematoma, caused by bleeding beneath the periosteum, is limited by suture lines. This swelling may take many weeks to disappear and frequently leaves a calcified ridge. Its resolution may be associated with an increased level of jaundice.

Other forms of haemorrhage are rare (see Fig. 35.2).

Fontanelles. Both the anterior and posterior should be easily palpable at birth. The posterior fontanelle closes by 10 weeks of age and the anterior fontanelle should have closed completely by 2 years of age.

Eyes.

1. Congenital cataracts occur secondary to intrauterine infection (particularly rubella), and galactosaemia.

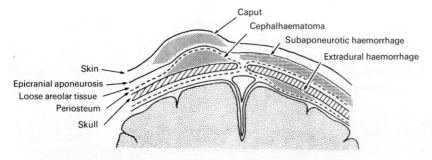

Fig. 35.2 Layers of the fetal skill illustrating possible sites of haemorrhage.

2. A *coloboma*, a defect extending from the iris through the aqueous and vitreous humours back to the retina, is associated with chromosomal abnormalities.

Face

The features associated with chromosomal abnormality, such as Down syndrome, may be obvious at first glance. Other major anomalies such as a cleft palate are not necessarily easily visible. Teeth may be present, commonly in the central incisor region and there is a familial pattern of occurrence. They should be removed in the newborn period to prevent aspiration.

Chest

The clavicles should be checked particularly if there has been any shoulder dystocia. Although callus formation occurs rapidly, a palpable lump will only appear after the infant is discharged from the maternity ward. Nevertheless, crepitus may be detected following delivery. No specific treatment is required. The apex beat should be palpated routinely in the 4th left intercostal space, midclavicular line. Isolated dextrocardia is associated with intracardiac anomalies, but total situs inversus, with the liver on the left, is associated with a normal heart. Flow murmurs are often heard in the newborn period.

Abdomen

The liver is just palpable in the newborn period. Normal kidneys are very difficult to palpate and the spleen is not palpable. Femoral pulses should be felt and their presence recorded. Absence of femoral pulses on discharge examination that were clearly felt on the labour ward may indicate a hypoplastic left heart.

Genitalia and anus

Hypospadias, with malposition of the urethral meatus is associated with a hooded prepuce and chordee, a tethering of the ventral penile shaft. In a term infant both testes are descended into a well formed scrotal sac. The female clitoris may look large in the first weeks of life. The anus should be checked for patency.

Hips

Congenital dislocation of the hip encompasses varying degrees of instability, subluxation and dysplasia of the hip joint. It occurs in one per thousand live births and is more common in girls, breech deliveries or in infants with a positive family history.

Skeletal system

Although the incidence of spina bifida is declining, it is important to inspect the back for any bony defect or hairy naevus before the infant leaves the delivery suite. Positional abnormalities of the foot are common but club foot (talipes) requiring intervention may occur in association with spina bifida or in association with previous amniocentesis and leakage of liquor.

CARE IN THE FIRST WEEK OF LIFE

Feeding

Most problems in the first week of life centre around feeding. Babies should be breast-fed for at least the first three months and can be put to the breast on the labour ward. Breast milk is the most easily digestible, clean and convenient milk available with protective effects against gastrointestinal infection in infancy and possibly atopy and asthma in childhood. Term babies will obtain 80% of the available milk in the first five minutes and therefore 15 minutes on each breast is more than adequate for their needs.

There are almost no contraindications to breast-feeding. Active tuberculosis in the mother is not a contraindication but infants should be protected with isoniazid and an isoniazid-resistant BCG. HIV-positive mothers should probably not breast-feed, at least in the Western world where commercial milks are readily available. Cytotoxic drug therapy in the mother remains the only absolute contraindication to breast feeding.

A wide variety of cow's milk and soya based formula feeds are available for those not wishing to breast-feed. The protein, calcium and phosphorous in these commercial milks have been reduced to similar levels to human breast milk. All commercial milks have a similar formulation, whatever the brand, and are fortified with vitamins and iron. The term baby, whether breast or bottle-fed, does not require vitamin or iron supplements. A term baby should receive fluid, whether it be 5% dextrose, sterile water or milk, within four hours of birth. On the first day, babies require 60 ml/kg/day increasing to 150 ml/kg/day by five days of age and for the first three months. Babies are usually fed 3–4 hourly at this time, so a baby weighing 3 kg requires 450 ml of milk per day and should take approximately 75 ml at each feed once feeding is established. All babies normally lose weight in the first week but should have regained their birth weight by 10 days of age. A loss of more than 10% of body weight in the first week is pathological.

Hygiene

Infants usually receive their first bath whilst on the postnatal wards, since this is a suitable place to teach mothers how to care for their babies. The timing of the first bath is immaterial. The umbilical cord requires no special care but should be kept clean and dry. Separation should have occurred by 10 days of age.

Routine tests

The Guthrie test (for phenylketonuria) is performed on all infants between 7 and 10 days of age, whether they are in hospital or at home. The infant must have been on milk feed for at least 24 hours and not taking antibiotics. Blood is taken by heel prick on to a card and sent for estimation of phenylalanine and TSH to exclude hypothyroidism.

PATHOLOGICAL EVENTS

Birth trauma

1. Caput succedaneum (see p. 295).
2. Cephalhaematoma (see p. 295).
3. Subaponeurotic haemorrhage (see p. 295) occasionally occurs in black babies. Blood loss into the soft tissue may be quite severe and result in hypotension and shock. The baby will have a boggy mass like a helmet surrounding the skull. Aspiration has no part to play but active resuscitation with replacement of the blood loss is life-saving. Bleeding within the skull into the extradural or subdural spaces is rare in modern obstetric practice.
4. Mechanical trauma. Direct mechanical trauma in the delivery of a large baby may result in an Erb's palsy with temporary paralysis of the cervical roots C5, C6 (Fig. 35.3). The affected arm is held in the characteristic 'waiter's tip' position. Klumpke's paralysis (arm flexed at elbow and wrist) affecting C7 and C8 and the intrinsic muscles of the hand is uncommon. Both recover spontaneously but physiotherapy is recommended. Forceps pressing on the outlet of the facial nerve may cause a temporary facial palsy. Traction on the head may tear fibres of the sternomastoid muscles and a palpable lump may be found on the contracted side. This may only be noticed after the first week. Physiotherapy is also recommended in this condition.

Minor sepsis

Sticky eyes

This is a common complaint in the newborn period. *Streptococcus, Staphylococcus* and *Haemophilus influenzae* are the usual pathogens and treatment is with neomycin cream. Chloramphenicol drops will mask *Chlamydia* as a

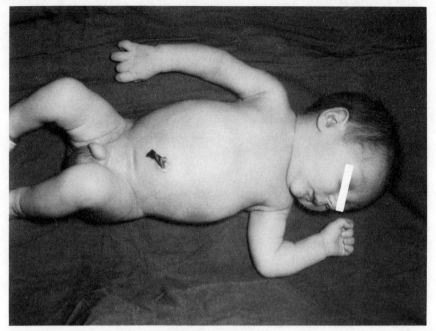

Fig. 35.3 Erb's palsy.

cause. *Chlamydia* is becoming increasingly common and should be treated with tetracycline eye drops and erythromycin orally. If gross purulent secretion is present, swabs for *Gonococcus* must be taken. Persistent sticky eyes may indicate a blocked tear duct.

Umbilical cord

The umbilical cord always becomes sticky and slightly offensive prior to separation. Routine cleaning is all that is required and separation occurs by 10 days. Organisms may be cultured from the stump but treatment is not required unless there is an umbilical flare and the baby is ill.

Skin sepsis

Paronychia and widespread septic spots caused by *Staphylococci* are common. Paronychia requires systemic antibiotic treatment. A few septic spots may be managed by antiseptic added to daily baths.

Jaundice

Babies frequently develop 'physiological' jaundice between the 2nd and 5th day of life. This is caused by immaturity of liver enzymes resulting in raised

Table 35.1 Common causes of jaundice.

Cause	Investigation
Extravascular blood	Physical examination
Rhesus incompatibility ABO incompatibility	Coombs' test, maternal blood group, infant blood group, anti-A or anti-B haemolysins in the mother
Infection	Urine for microscopy, culture and sensitivity. Full blood count, blood cultures, lumbar puncture, chest X-ray
Metabolic disease	Blood glucose, blood bicarbonate, G6PD levels, urine for reducing substances
Prolonged jaundice Hypothyroidism	TSH, T4
Biliary atresia	Ultrasound scan of the liver

levels of unconjugated bilirubin. Higher levels of bilirubin may be seen in babies who are dehydrated or who have marked bruising or a cephal-haematoma at delivery. There is said to be an increased incidence of jaundice in breast-fed babies, the so-called 'breast milk jaundice', but it is unclear whether this is a true clinical entity or not. No specific treatment is required for mild jaundice.

Jaundice detectable within the first 24 hours or levels of unconjugated bilirubin above 270 mmol/litre require further investigation and treatment. Common causes of jaundice and prolonged jaundice are listed in Table 35.1.

Treatment

Phototherapy using the blue part of the light spectrum decreases the level of bilirubin in the blood. No long-term detrimental effects have been documented from its use although the infant's eyes should be protected from the light. Infants are given 20 ml/kg/day above their fluid requirements whilst they are jaundiced.

Table 35.2 Common causes of fits.

Cause	Investigation
Hypoglycaemia	BM Stix, blood sugar
Hypocalcaemia	Blood calcium level
Birth trauma	Skull X-ray
Congenital structural abnormality	Ultrasound of the head, CT scan
Asphyxia	Blood pH, urea and electrolytes
Meningitis	Lumbar puncture

High levels of unconjugated bilirubin (above 400 mmol in the normal term infant) may result in selective damage to the basal ganglia (kernicterus). The infant develops sensorineural deafness and athetoid cerebral palsy. The danger is particularly great in infants where there has been associated asphyxia. Exchange transfusion, removing the high levels of unconjugated bilirubin from the circulation, will prevent this serious complication.

Fits

See Table 35.2.

Treatment

Diazemul 0.25 mg/kg given intravenously will control fits initially. If they are caused by hypoglycaemia, 0.5 ml/kg of 50% dextrose should be given intravenously.

Renal abnormalities

The introduction of antenatal ultrasound has made the detection of structural renal abnormalities in the fetus a common event. Such infants require confirmatory ultrasound postnatally and prophylactic antibiotics should be given to prevent any possible urinary tract infection until the results of the postnatal ultrasound are available. It is very important to prevent septicaemia and scarring of the kidneys in the newborn period.

THE PRETERM INFANT

Assessment and management

Delivery

All infants under 28 weeks' gestation should be delivered in a regional centre or transferred as soon as possible after birth. Infants between 28 and 32 weeks' gestation with normal lungs can safely be managed in a district special care baby unit if appropriate trained nursing and medical staff are both available. Infants with respiratory distress at this gestation should be transferred to an intensive care unit. Most infants above 32 weeks' gestation can safely be managed in the district hospital.

Labour ward

Asphyxia of the preterm infant should be prevented if respiratory distress and intraventricular haemorrhage or hypoxic brain damage are to be

Table 35.3 Admission to a special care baby unit.

Justifiable reasons for admission	Unjustifiable reasons for routine admission
Birth-weight less than 2.0 kg	Complicated delivery (forceps, ventouse, breech, LSCS)
Gestational age less than 35 weeks	Mild birth asphyxia
Respiratory distress	Meconium stained liquor
Severe jaundice	Multiple pregnancy
Convulsions	Adverse previous history
	Small for gestational age
	Jittery
	Mild jaundice
	Minor feeding problem
	Social problem

avoided. Infants should be rapidly resuscitated immediately after birth and transferred to a special care baby unit.

The prognosis of premature infants is highly dependent on the adequacy of the initial resuscitation. A fetus less than 24 weeks' gestation has very little chance of survival in a district hospital and resuscitation is not appropriate. Between 24 and 28 weeks' gestation, resuscitation should be offered immediately and the baby assessed on the labour ward. If there is a poor response to resuscitation, the eyelids are fused or there is gross bruising, the outlook is poor and further treatment may then be withdrawn. After 28 weeks' gestation the fetus is legally viable and full treatment must be offered.

Special care baby unit (SCBU)

On arrival in SCBU the infant is weighed, the head circumference is recorded and routine swabs from the ear (where amniotic fluid collects) and the umbilicus are taken. A gastric aspirate is sent for microscopy and culture since this is a good early indicator of infection from amniotic fluid.

A BM Stix is recorded and fluid is given as soon as possible either nasogastrically or by an intravenous infusion if the baby is unwell. In the sick preterm infant, an arterial gas is taken to assess the level of acidosis which also provides a good indicator of birth asphyxia.

The gestational age of an infant is estimated by the so-called 'Dubowitz' assessment which depends on a combination of the baby's neurological behaviour with physical characteristics to give an estimation of gestational age independent of birth weight. This is useful when maternal dates are doubtful or when the infant is of unexpectedly low birth-weight. In such a case an infant may be identified as being small for gestational age but mature, or preterm and appropriate weight for gestation, or both.

Infants under 1.8 kg require nursing in an incubator to maintain a neutral thermal environment in which they can grow. They find it difficult to maintain their body temperature in a cot. Infants above this weight are frequently put in an incubator to be observed for at least the first 24 hours.

Preterm or small for gestational age infants are prone to hypoglycaemia. Normal glucose levels in the newborn period are 2–4 mmol/l. Levels of blood sugar below this may result in apnoea, fits and lasting brain damage. Early feeding is essential. Infants below 35 weeks' gestation are unlikely to be able to suck adequately and will need some nasogastric feeds. There are doubts as to whether breast milk is the appropriate feed for an extremely low birth-weight baby and preterm formula feeds are available.

PATHOLOGICAL EVENTS

Apnoea. Immaturity of the brain stem often leads to irregular respiratory effort in the preterm infant. This can be treated satisfactorily with theophylline orally or rectally. Respiratory distress, infection, hypoglycaemia, convulsions and drugs may also result in apnoea and these causes should be excluded.

Respiratory Distress Syndrome (RDS)

Anatomy and physiology. Although Type 1 and Type 2 pneumocytes are present, the final subdivision of the lung into alveoli occurs after 24 weeks and only air saccules are present. Alveoli form at 28 weeks. For this maturation to occur, the fetus must breath in utero and liquid must be present in the lungs.

Pathophysiology

Exomphalos.

The surfactant lining, which is essential for lung compliance, is only produced by the type 2 pneumocytes from 24 weeks' gestation onwards. The factors predisposing to delayed production or increased reabsorption and therefore the development of respiratory distress syndrome are:

1. Preterm delivery
2. Male sex
3. Hypoxia
4. Hypercapnia
5. Acidosis
6. Hypothermia
7. Hypoglycaemia
8. Caesarean section
9. Second twin
10. Intraventricular haemorrhage
11. Hypotension
12. Infant of a diabetic mother.

Conditions associated with lung hypoplasia

Prolonged oligohydramnios

1. Renal agenesis or severe dysplasia
2. Obstruction of lower urinary tract
3. Prolonged rupture of membranes
4. Amniocentesis followed by leakage of liquor.

Skeletal dysplasias

1. Thanatrophic dwarfism
2. Lethal variant of osteogenesis imperfecta.

Anomalies affecting the diaphragm

1. Congenital diaphragmatic hernia
2. Severe congenital muscle disorders.

Damage to the CNS

Anencephaly.

Clinical features of RDS

1. A respiratory rate above the normal value of 40 breaths per minute
2. Use of accessory muscles of respiration
3. Flaring nostrils
4. Grunting.

Treatment. An increase in ambient humidified oxygen is always necessary. If this is ineffective or the baby is developing apnoea, ventilatory support may be required.

Intraventricular haemorrhage (IVH)

A layer of capillaries, the so-called germinal layer, spreads over the caudate nucleus in infants less than 32 weeks' gestation. This layer disappears with increasing maturity so that bleeding from the germinal layer into the ventricle, an intraventricular haemorrhage, becomes increasingly rare after 32 weeks. The introduction of real time ultrasound through the fontanelle has shown that minor forms of IVH are common in the preterm infant and are not necessarily associated with handicap. Bleeding that fills the ventricles (grade 3 IVH) or goes into brain substance (grade 4 IVH) is likely to lead to hydrocephalus or a hemiparesis.

The consequences of preterm delivery

The increased survival of very small infants has not led to an increase in the proportion of handicapped babies in the general population but clearly such babies are particularly prone to such problems.

Deafness

Middle ear disease is common in all children, particularly the preterm. Damage to the auditory central pathways may also occur as a result of anoxia, antibiotics or even incubator noise.

Blindness

Proliferation of small vessels in the retina spreading through the vitreous humour resulting in retinal detachment may occur in the preterm infant exposed to high levels of oxygen. This may lead to blindness. Squints are also common in the preterm infant.

Respiratory problems

Bronchopulmonary dysplasia or lung fibrosis resulting from the combination of infection, high inspired oxygen levels and barotrauma from ventilators is a common sequel of long-term ventilation. Affected infants may develop cor pulmonale and have an increased admission rate to hospital with chest infections in the first two years of life.

Neurological damage

Cerebral palsy is defined as a motor disorder present at the time of delivery. It is not progressive but clearly its effects may become more marked as the child grows. Since the primary cause is usually hypoxia there is a high association with developmental delay.

SMALL FOR GESTATIONAL AGE (SGA) INFANTS

Definition

Infants whose weight is below the 10th centile for their gestational age.

Interesting facts

In Great Britain 7% of all babies are of low birth-weight ($< 2.5\,$kg). A third of these infants are small for gestational age.

Aetiology

Slowing of growth usually occurs in the third trimester. If growth retardation occurs in the second trimester, intrauterine infection or chromosomal abnormalities should be excluded. Hypertension accounts for 35% of all growth retarded infants. Most SGA infants are asymmetrically growth retarded with preservation of head growth and body length at the expense of weight.

DELIVERY

SGA infants withstand asphyxia badly and the presence or absence of birth asphyxia is the biggest determinant of long-term handicap.

PROBLEMS IN THE FIRST WEEK OF LIFE

1. *Hypothermia.* SGA infants have a large head and less body fat and are at particular risk from heat loss.
2. *Hypoglycaemia.* Results from inadequate glycogen stores, impaired gluconeogenesis and increased circulating insulin levels.
3. *PCV.* May be raised due to relative intrauterine hypoxia. This increased blood viscosity can lead to cerebral thrombosis.

Treatment

Early feeding and regular BM Stix monitoring in the first 48 hours is essential. Feeds should be formula or breast milk but, if the stix falls below 2 mmol/litre another feed should be given via a nasogastric tube. If the baby has symptoms such as apnoea, jitteriness or convulsions, then an intravenous bolus of 50% dextrose 0.5 ml/kg stat is given followed by a 10% dextrose infusion.

Outcome

There is epidemiological evidence that term SGA infants are at risk of minimal cerebral dysfunction with an increase in clumsiness, hyperactivity, speech and language problems. This is even more likely to occur in the preterm SGA infant, particularly if there is associated birth asphyxia.

36. Sexually transmitted diseases

S. E. Barton

Expectations of the examiners

The candidate will be expected to understand the general principles of the management of sexually transmitted diseases (STD). These include the following:

1. Appropriate history taking and clinical examination.
2. Where possible, the relevant tests to obtain a microbiological diagnosis should be performed before therapy is commenced.
3. The finding of any STD suggests that others may also have been acquired. As several conditions may be totally asymptomatic (e.g. cervical gonorrhoea or chlamydial infection, latent syphilis, vaginal condylomata acuminata), it is essential that both clinical examination and laboratory investigations are extensive enough to screen for a wide range of infectious agents.
4. The diagnosis and treatment of STD should include advice and education of the patient as well as contact tracing of her partners. This will help to prevent her reinfection after treatment, as well as reduce the reservoir of infection within the community. Often the presentation of a woman with a suspected STD will provide a valuable opportunity for her to receive advice about contraception.

It is essential that the candidate has a clear understanding of which clinical conditions can be managed by general practitioners, and which should be referred to departments of genitourinary medicine or gynaecology for specialist assessment and therapy.

Definition

A major problem with producing a satisfactory definition of an STD is that certain STDs produce an entirely local genital infection (e.g. trichomoniasis, genital warts) whereas others may cause severe systemic disease (e.g. secondary syphilis, AIDS). Moreover, not all STD are *always* transmitted by sexual contact (e.g. vertical transmission of congenital syphilis or HIV infection) and the question of whether to include conditions which are associated with sexual activity, but not necessarily transmitted, such as bacterial vaginosis, is a vexed one. To avoid such problems, this chapter could be retitled 'Genital and systemic diseases of women, resulting from infections which can be transmitted sexually'!

Interesting facts

Women with STD present with four main clinical conditions. These are vaginal discharge, pelvic inflammatory disease, genital lesions (ulceration or condylomata), and systemic infections. Individual infectious agents can cause disease in more than one of these categories and most can also be asymptomatic.

This chapter will consider each of these broad clinical categories in turn, describing the common causes of each and their management.

VAGINAL DISCHARGE

Pathophysiology

The normal vaginal secretions of a premenopausal adult woman consist of desquamated vaginal epithelial cells, vaginal wall transudate, cervical mucus secretions, a variable volume of fluid from the upper genital tract and microorganisms (mainly Döderlein's lactobacilli). There is an individual and often cyclical variation in the amount of these secretions, as well as considerable variation in different women's perceptions of what constitutes a 'normal discharge'.

Aetiology

The causes of an alteration in vaginal discharge are summarized in Table 36.1. Several of these may coexist, for instance a woman who has recently commenced sexual activity may also have begun to take the pill, have vaginal candidiasis and tried douching with antiseptics to treat this. Such cases mean that accurate history taking, careful clinical examination and obtaining suitable specimens for laboratory tests are essential to make a correct diagnosis.

Non-infectious causes of alterations in vaginal discharge include the hormonal changes which occur at puberty and the menopause, as well as changes during the menstrual cycle. Retained foreign objects usually present with an offensive vaginal discharge, with the cause often being a piece of tampon. Chemical vaginitis usually occurs with the use of antiseptic douches, but also as a reaction to the use of perfumed or disinfectant bath additives. Non-infectious, gynaecological causes are less common and include genital tract neoplasms, vaginal fistulae and uterine prolapse.

The commonest infectious cause of a symptomatic vaginal discharge is

Table 36.1 Aetiology of altered vaginal discharge.

Non-infectious
Physiological
    Puberty
    Menstrual cycle
    Sexual activity
    Pregnancy
    Menopause

Pathological
    Foreign body
    Chemical vaginitis
    Drug-related
    Gynaecological

Infectious
Vaginal
    Candida albicans
    Trichomonas vaginalis
    Bacterial vaginosis
    Others
        Human papillomavirus
        β haemolytic streptococcus

Cervical
    Neisseria gonorrhoeae
    Chlamydia trachomatis
    Herpes simplex virus

---

the yeast, *Candida albicans*. More than 50 000 cases of vaginal candidiasis are treated in STD clinics annually in the UK. In a small percentage of cases, other candidal species or *Torulopsis glabrata* may be the yeast involved, but the clinical picture is similar. Another frequently identified cause is *Trichomonas vaginalis*, a flagellated protozoon, which accounts for 25% of cases of vaginal discharge in the USA.

In the considerable number of women who present with vaginal discharge, but have no evidence of either of these infections, a diagnosis of bacterial vaginosis is often made, however a specific aetiological agent has not been identified for this condition (see below). Rarer causes of vaginal discharge include streptococcal infection or that associated with extensive vulvovaginal warts (although this is often due to secondary infection).

Infection of the columnar epithelium of the endocervix by *Neisseria gonorrhoeae* or *Chlamydia trachomatis* (serotypes D–K) can result in vaginal discharge alone, or be complicated by pelvic pain and systemic symptoms, or be completely asymptomatic (see Pelvic inflammatory disease). Herpes simplex virus (HSV) infection may produce a vaginal discharge secondary to cervical lesions during a primary or recurrent episode; indeed, it is important to note that cervical and vaginal HSV lesions can occur in the absence of any externally visible, vulval lesions (see Genital lesions).

Assessment

Points in the history which may suggest particular infectious causes of an increased vaginal discharge include the following:

1. Pregnancy, diabetes mellitus, immunosuppression, recent antibiotic treatment, itchy vulval irritation or dyspareunia suggest candidiasis.
2. New sexual partner, copious irritant discharge and malodour suggest trichomoniasis.
3. Presence of an IUCD, malodorous vaginal discharge and dyspareunia suggest bacterial vaginosis. However, as no specific historical features are pathognomonic for any particular infection, clinical examination is essential.
4. Vulvovaginal erythema and oedema, vulval excoriation and the presence of curdy discharge with white/yellow plaques suggest candidiasis.
5. Excessive, often frothy yellow/green malodorous discharge suggests trichomoniasis.
6. Thin, adherent, homogenous, grey/white, offensive smelling discharge suggests bacterial vaginosis.

Despite these typical appearances, reliance on clinical diagnosis will often be misleading or miss the presence of multiple infections.

Investigations

A vaginal smear on a microscope slide can be Gram-stained to demonstrate typical Gram-positive ovoid spores or tubular pseudo-hyphae of *Candida albicans*. Sabouraud's media can be inoculated to provide culture confirmation.

A drop of discharge on a slide, suspended in saline under a cover slip, can be examined as a wet mount preparation. This may reveal the presence of motile, flagellated trichomonads. Although this is a very reliable method of diagnosing trichomoniasis, this can be confirmed by using Whittington–Feinberg culture medium.

The diagnosis of bacterial vaginosis is based on the finding of typical 'clue cells' in a Gram-stained vaginal smear. These are characteristically granular epithelial cells, with coccobacillary organisms attached to their surface giving a 'salt and pepper appearance'. In addition, the vaginal discharge will have a pH > 5 and release a characteristic 'fishy' odour on mixing with 10% KOH. The pH of vaginal discharge is also raised in trichomoniasis, but is usually < 4.5 in cases of candidal infection; this can be a quick and helpful guide to diagnosis. Ideally though, all women with vaginal discharge should have a full set of microbiological tests performed on vaginal and cervical (to exclude gonococcal and chlamydial infection) specimens.

Treatment

Vaginal candidiasis may be treated topically using an imidazole derivative, such as clotrimazole (500 mg × 1 or 200 mg × 3 nocte) or econazole (150 mg × 1 or × 3 nocte). These may be administered as vaginal creams or pessaries and will produce a cure in over 90% of cases. Recently, orally administered, 'one-day' therapies (e.g. fluconazole and itraconazole) have become available. These are claimed to be preferred by patients and to reduce the incidence of recurrent infections. However, their expense currently limits their use to recurrent cases.

Metronidazole (400 mg b.d. for 5 days) is the treatment of choice for both trichomoniasis and bacterial vaginosis.

As *T. vaginalis* has been found to infect the male urethra and cause some cases of non-specific urethritis (NSU), it is important that the male partners of infected women are treated to prevent reinfection. However, there is less evidence to support such contact tracing for cases of candidiasis and bacterial vaginosis; this is only usually performed in cases of recurrent infection. Indeed, a further problem lies in the high prevalence of apparently asymptomatic women with laboratory evidence of these two conditions. Whilst further research is awaited into the local immune responses to candidal carriage and the role of *Gardnerella vaginalis* and anaerobes in bacterial vaginosis, most authorities do not advocate treating asymptomatic women.

All women with vaginal discharge should also be given simple advice on wearing looser cotton underwear, avoiding irritant soaps or bath additives and general health information.

SUMMARY

Vaginal discharge is a common presenting complaint which merits a proper clinical assessment and accurate diagnosis to ensure the correct management.

PELVIC INFLAMMATORY DISEASE (PID)

Definition

PID is an infection of the endometrium, fallopian tubes and/or contiguous structures which is usually attributed to the ascent of microorganisms via the cervix and vagina.

Interesting facts

It is estimated that nearly 100 000 women in the UK develop PID each year. After one episode of infection, 12.8% of women will suffer from tubal infertility; after three episodes, this figure rises to 75%. In addition, chronic pelvic pain, dyspareunia, pelvic adhesions and an increased subsequent risk of ectopic pregnancy add to the morbidity associated with this condition.

Pathophysiology

It is unknown why only 10% of women with gonococcal or chlamydial cervical infection will develop PID. The barriers to the ascent of microorganisms include cervical mucus, which forms a mechanical barrier in the narrow endocervical canal, as well as containing lysozyme and immunoglobulins (especially IgA). Cyclical menstrual shedding of the endometrium may also contribute to preventing the establishment of uterine infection. In addition, the uterotubal junction as well as the downward flow of tubal mucus also appear to act as further mechanical barriers to ascending infection.

Except in the few cases where infection is spread intra-abdominally (e.g. from an infected appendix), all of these barriers have to be passed by an ascending pathogen. This is often precipitated by trauma to the cervix and uterus as occurs in spontaneous and induced abortions, childbirth, or surgical procedures, especially the insertion of an IUCD. There is some evidence that spermatozoa and the motile protozoon, *Trichomonas vaginalis*, may play a role in carrying *N. gonorrhoeae*, *C. trachomatis* or other microorganisms, into the upper genital tract. Once infected by one organism, the local damage to the fallopian tubes may result in an increased susceptibility to infection by other microorganisms, such as anaerobes and coliforms.

Aetiology

The question of whether PID is caused by a single or multiple infectious agents is unanswered. The current consensus view is that most commonly *N. gonorrhoeae* or *C. trachomatis* (types D–K) initiate an attack, but are often replaced by later opportunistic bacterial invaders, such as the anaerobic species *Peptococcus* and *Bacteroides*. The detection of *Mycoplasma hominis, Ureaplasma urealyticum* and even herpes simplex virus from the fallopian tubes of women with PID has implicated these agents as pathogens, but further evidence is awaited. Finally, it is important that pelvic tuberculosis is not forgotten as an occasional cause of PID. It rarely presents as an acute infection nowadays, but it is essential to exclude it as a cause of infertility and pelvic pain, especially in women from high-risk groups.

Assessment

The spectrum of symptoms and signs present in cases of PID is very wide, and although bilateral low abdominal pain and an increased vaginal discharge are common presentations, no clinical picture is reliable. Because of this, gynaecologists will only make an accurate clinical diagnosis of PID in two-thirds of cases. This may be partly improved by using strict diagnostic criteria:

1. Abdominal tenderness, with or without rebound tenderness
2. Cervical motion tenderness ('excitation')
3. Adnexal tenderness.

All three must be present with at least one of the following:

1. Gram-negative intracellular diplococci seen on microscopy of endo-cervical secretions
2. Fever > 38°C
3. Leucocytosis > 10 000/mm³
4. Purulent material in peritoneum on laparoscopy or culdocentesis
5. Pelvic abscess on clinical examination or ultrasound.

The inaccuracy in clinical diagnosis of PID, as well as the potentially fatal error of missing important differential conditions such as ectopic pregnancy, has lead some authors to recommend that all women with pelvic pain should have a diagnostic laparoscopy performed. However, few centres have facilities for this and most will only perform laparoscopy on the most severe cases or those who do not respond to 48–72 hours of antibiotic therapy. Early laparoscopy allows the microbiological sampling of the peritoneum and tubal fimbriae which may give a more accurate guide to the causative organisms than samples from the vagina or cervix.

Investigations

In all cases of suspected PID, endocervical swabs should be taken for culture of *N. gonorrhoeae* and the detection of *C. trachomatis* (by culture, ELISA or microimmunofluorescence tests). The addition of a urethral swab will increase the sensitivity of detecting *N. gonorrhoeae*. High vaginal swabs are only useful for the detection of associated candidiasis, tricho-moniasis or other vaginal infections. A full blood count and differential white cell count should be performed. Serum should be grouped and saved for all patients who may need a laparoscopy.

As part of the investigations to exclude other differential diagnoses in women with acute pelvic pain, a midstream specimen of urine for microscopy and culture, a pregnancy test and an ultrasound examination are often indicated.

Treatment

Bed rest and adequate analgesia are essential. Initial antibiotic therapy should be active against the range of pathogens commonly implicated in

PID. As no single agent is suitable for this purpose, a combination of the following is suitable:

1. For *N. gonorrhoeae*: oral ampicillin 3.5 g and probenecid 1 g stat or if high risk of penicillinase producing (PPNG) strains, use either spectinomycin 2 g i.m. stat or ciprofloxacin 250 mg orally stat
2. For *C. trachomatis*: doxycycline 100 mg b.d. or erythromycin 500 mg q.d.s. for 14 days
3. For anaerobes: metronidazole 400 mg b.d. for 7 days.

The most important component of outpatient therapy is the need for regular reassessment every 2–3 days to assess the clinical response to treatment.

In hospitalized patients, a broad spectrum agent such as gentamicin 80 mg i.v. 8-hourly is often added to a parenteral version of the above regimen. Women with severe cases of PID (i.e. febrile with generalized abdominal tenderness) need admission to hospital as well as those in whom the diagnosis is uncertain, those unable to tolerate oral therapy, those who do not respond to oral therapy and those with suspected complications such as tubovarian abscesses.

In addition to treatment of the patient herself, it is essential that her recent sexual partners are examined and treated for evidence of STD. One study found that 68% of the partners of women with chlamydial PID had evidence of urethritis, as did 12% of partners of women without *Chlamydia* detected.

SUMMARY

The clinical diagnosis of PID is often inaccurate. Especially if a diagnostic laparoscopy is not performed, it is essential that endocervical specimens for *N. gonorrhoeae* and *C. trachomatis* are taken prior to commencing appropriate antibiotic therapy. By earlier and more accurate diagnosis, frequent clinical reassessment and contact tracing of sexual partners, the severe morbidity of PID might be reduced.

GENITAL LESIONS

GENITAL ULCERATION

Interesting facts

Genital HSV infection is the STD which has shown the greatest rise in incidence in the past decade. Recent evidence from Africa has suggested that genital ulceration may be an important factor in the transmission of human immunodeficiency virus (HIV) infection. Whether this will be an important factor in heterosexual transmission of HIV in Europe and North America remains to be seen.

Table 36.2 Differential diagnosis of genital ulceration.

Non-infectious
Physical or chemical trauma
Erythema multiforme
Stevens–Johnson syndrome
Behçets disease
Lichen planus
Crohn's disease
Vulval malignancy

Infectious
Herpes simplex virus
1° or 2° syphilis
Lymphogranuloma venereum
Granuloma inguinale
Varicella zoster
Scabies/pediculosis pubis

Pathophysiology/aetiology (see Table 36.2)

Although recurrent genital HSV infection is often a mild and self-limiting condition, primary episodes may be severe and require hospital admission. Most genital infections are due to HSV type 2, but up to 20% of cases are caused by type 1, which usually infects the perioral area. A primary attack occurs in patients with no previous exposure to type 1 or 2, who lack any neutralizing antibody: these are usually the cases with extensive genital lesions and severe systemic complications. In those who have previously acquired neutralizing antibody, usually via a perioral HSV type 1 infection, the 'first episode' genital infection is usually milder.

The frequency and severity of recurrent HSV infections is worse in patients infected by HSV type 2 and in those patients with immunosuppression. However, the cause of the wide variation in rates of recurrences amongst otherwise healthy individuals is being increasingly attributed to psychoneuroimmunological factors.

Assessment

Careful history taking of any previous episodes, a typical prodrome of itching, dysuria, painful groins and legs and blistering prior to ulceration strongly suggest recurrent HSV infection. The use of new soaps or antiseptics, recent drug ingestion, previous dermatological problems and recent foreign travel as well as a full sexual history, are all also important.

Clinical examination must include thorough inspection of the lower genital tract and perianal region, as well as a general physical examination with a diligent search for lymphadenopathy or coexistent oropharyngeal lesions or other skin rashes.

In the UK, painful genital ulceration is usually herpetic in origin whereas

Table 36.3   Syphilis serology; time from exposure to positivity.

Fluorescent treponemal antibody test (FTA)	3–4 weeks
Venereal diseases research laboratory (VDRL) test	3–5 weeks
Treponema pallidum haemagglutination assay (TPHA)	8–10 weeks

painless ulcers are syphilitic: solitary ulceration suggesting a 1° chancre and multiple ulcers occurring in 2° syphilis. However, as these infections can and do coexist it is essential that tests for both are performed on women with genital ulceration.

Unless there is a high level of clinical awareness and a good light in the examination room, the detection of the ectoparasites which cause pediculosis pubis or scabies will be missed. In the former, *Phthirus pubis* ('crabs') themselves, or their eggs ('nits') are visibly attached to the base of pubic hairs and in the latter, if the typical burrows of the scabies mite are lifted with a needle and the contents placed in 10% KOH on a slide, *Sarcoptes scabiei* may be visualized on microscopy.

Investigations

All new cases of genital ulcers should have samples taken for viral culture of HSV. If facilities exist, a specimen of serum expressed from the ulcer should be obtained and examined by dark ground microscopy to search for the live organisms of *Treponema pallidum*. Whether this is done or not, it is mandatory to obtain a venous blood sample for syphilis serology, which should be repeated six weeks later in cases of a suspected 1° chancre. The times of appearance of positive serological tests for syphilis are shown in Table 36.3.

The Venereal Disease Research Laboratory (VDRL) test is a non-specific test which is often used in conjunction with the TPHA in screening antenatal patients for syphilis. It can be complicated by a biological false positive reaction following acute viral infections, typhoid or yellow fever immunizations and autoimmune conditions such as disseminated lupus erythematosus and rheumatoid arthritis. Thus it is essential that any positive test is repeated and combined with clinical examination before any treatment is commenced. In patients with a history of overseas travel or sexual contacts from the third world, it may be indicated to take cultures for *Haemophilus ducreyi*, a Gram-negative facultative anaerobe which causes chancroid and blood for serological diagnosis of *Lymphogranuloma venereum*, which is caused by *Chlamydia trachomatis* serotypes L_1, L_2 and L_3.

It is essential that a full screen for other STD is obtained from all patients who present with genital ulceration, which is usually best performed in departments of genitourinary medicine.

Treatment

Primary and first episode cases of genital HSV infection should be treated with systemic acyclovir, a viral DNA polymerase inhibitor. This is administered as either 200 mg 5× daily orally for five days or via intravenous infusion in severe cases. This will diminish the symptoms and new ulcer formation as well as reduce the risk of complications such as urinary retention occurring. This latter complication should be managed by analgesia, urinating into a warm bath, local anaesthesia and, only if all else fails, suprapubic catheterization.

In recurrent HSV infection, most patients will be able to tolerate 2–3 annual episodes of slight genital discomfort with simple measures, such as saline bathing, wearing loose underwear and avoiding sexual contact until the lesions have healed. However, in cases where the attacks are very frequent (> 1 per month), severely painful or in those patients suffering extreme psychosexual problems because of their HSV recurrences, continuous prophylactic acyclovir (200 mg orally q.d.s.) may be prescribed as suppressive therapy. Despite its low toxicity, it is essential that women receiving acyclovir use adequate contraception, as it is not yet licensed for use in pregnancy.

Syphilis should be treated by aqueous procaine penicillin 600 000 units/day, intramuscularly, for 15–20 days, or in patients allergic to penicillin, by a 30-day course of erythromycin or oxytetracycline (500 mg q.d.s. orally). Patients with primary and secondary syphilis should be warned of the Jarisch–Herxheimer reaction, a self-limiting febrile illness (thought to be related to the release of treponemal toxins and immune complex formation) which may be lessened by oral aspirin therapy. However, as more serious complications of therapy can occur in patients with later stages of cardiovascular or neurosyphilis, such cases should only be treated as inpatients under medical supervision. Although contact tracing is desirable in new cases of genital HSV infection, for syphilis this is mandatory and patients should be referred to the health adviser at the local GU medicine clinic to facilitate this, as well as the appropriate serological follow-up of the index patient.

Scabies and pediculosis pubis should be treated by 25% benzyl benzoate or 1% gamma benzene hexachloride applications from the neck downwards. Sexual partners and close family contacts should be seen and also treated.

Summary

Genital ulceration is an increasingly common problem in the UK. The range of disease extends from microscopic, solitary painless ulcers to multiple, severely painful systemic disease. Whatever the presentation, the correct diagnosis will only be obtained by careful clinical investigation and appropriate follow-up.

GENITAL CONDYLOMATA

Pathophysiology/aetiology

Genital condylomata acuminata (warts) are caused by human papilloma-virus (HPV). The lesions produced range from large exophytic warts (often types 6 and 11) to flat subclinical lesions (often types 16 and 18) which are only visible on colposcopic examination. All epithelia in the lower genital tract may be infected by HPV, often by multiple types. HPV types 16 and 18 infection of the cervical epithelium has been strongly implicated in the aetiology of cervical neoplasia. A less convincing association has also been proposed between vaginal and vulval HPV infection and premalignant conditions at these sites (VAIN and VIN). In view of the association of HPV with CIN, it has been recommended that women with a history of genital warts should have more frequent cervical cytology performed (i.e. annually), however, recent evidence suggests that the prevalence of CIN in women with a history of warts is no different to that found in women with any other STD.

The main differential diagnoses of genital warts are from molluscum contagiosum, caused by a pox virus, and condylomata lata, the classical lesions of secondary syphilis. Occasionally benign skin tags, sebaceous cysts or pigmented naevi can also confuse the diagnosis.

Assessment

A history of slow growing, painless, vulvovaginal lumps is highly sug-gestive of genital warts. This is one of the few STD to be diagnosed solely from their clinical appearance. However, a third of women who present with genital warts will have another STD present on more detailed investi-gation.

The lesions of molluscum contagiosum are also characteristic, being pearly white, umbilicated papules which may also be found on other parts of the body; they are transmitted by close, but not always sexual, contact.

Condylomata lata are coalescent, large fleshy masses of the papular lesions of 2° syphilis found in moist body areas. Other signs of 2° syphilis are usually present.

Investigations

A thorough examination of the lower genital tract, using a colposcope if available, is necessary to document the distribution of HPV infection present. A cervical cytology smear and a full screen for other STD should be performed.

In cases of 2° syphilis, dark ground examination of a smear from the condylomata lata will reveal spirochaetes and serological tests will be positive.

Treatment

External genital warts can be treated by chemical (25% podophyllin or trichloroacetic acid, washed off after 4 hours) or physical destruction (cryocautery, diathermy, laser). Internal warts should only be treated by physical methods due to the increased risk of side-effects with chemical agents, such as local ulceration and systemic absorption of podophyllin causing peripheral neuropathy and hypokalaemia. Moreover, podophyllin must be avoided in pregnancy due to the high risk of teratogenicity.

All methods have shown initial cure rates of between 70–90%, but whatever method is used, the long-term recurrence rates approach 50%. Although immunostimulants (e.g. isoprinosine, α interferon) have been tried as adjuvants to local therapy, it is unclear whether they are of long term benefit.

The value of contact tracing the male partners of women with genital warts serves to screen them for HPV and other STD, but also to reduce the risk of reinfection of the woman after treatment. The value of condom use by the male partner during, and for some time after, treatment has been suggested, but there is little evidence for this.

Molluscum contagiosum is treated by either applying neat phenol on a wooden stick into the centre of each lesion, or by using cryotherapy or electrocautery.

Summary

Genital warts often serve as a marker for other STD. As no systemic anti-HPV agent exists, the treatment is local. Long-term cure rates are often poor. Genital HPV infection, like other STD, acts as a risk factor for the development of cervical neoplasia; hence regular cervical cytological sampling of all women with warts, or any other STD, must be recommended.

ASYMPTOMATIC/SYSTEMIC

Aetiology

The three important systemic infections which may be sexually transmitted are syphilis, hepatitis B and HIV infection. All of these have asymptomatic phases in their natural history, all may be transmitted vertically by a pregnant woman and all may be fatal.

Assessment

Although each of these infections does produce well described clinical syndromes, the initial infection and subsequent carriage may be completely asymptomatic. Thus, the diagnosis of these infections will often be missed unless serological screening is performed in patients presenting with another STD. It is important that the patient understands the nature of any screening test performed and is counselled before the result is known.

Investigations

Hepatitis B may only be diagnosed by serology. Within 4–12 weeks of infection, hepatitis B surface (HBsAg) and e antigens (HBeAg) appear in the serum. HBsAg is usually cleared by four months from the onset of the infection and this usually precedes the appearance of anti-HBsAg, the antibody which confers long-term immunity. During this serological window, anti-hepatitis B core antibody may be the only positive indication of infection. HBeAg is usually cleared rapidly unless a chronic carrier state develops. Liver enzymes must be checked at regular intervals, but no pattern is pathognomonic of hepatitis B virus infection.

Seroconversion for anti-HIV typically occurs 4–12 weeks after acute infection, although longer delays have been described. The earlier detection of HIV p24 antigen (within 3 weeks of infection) or anti-HIV IgM in the serum may be useful in special cases (e.g. following a rape, a needlestick injury or during pregnancy). All positive tests should be repeated, along with a full screen for other STD, a full blood count and CD4 lymphocyte count.

Treatment

Acute viral hepatitis B is usually self-limiting and management is usually supportive. Advice on a low fat, high energy diet, the avoidance of alcohol and bed rest is given and the patient's liver enzymes regularly checked until normal. In chronic hepatitis, recent advances in antiviral therapy are promising. The contacts of patients who are infectious for hepatitis B should be seen and tested; immunization should be offered to the non-immune. Vaccination against hepatitis B infection should be offered to all non-immune patients in high-risk groups (e.g. prostitutes) and is essential for all medical, nursing and laboratory staff who come into contact with patients or their blood.

The management of asymptomatic patients with HIV infection is predominantly supportive, although prophylactic therapy against opportunistic infections and antiretroviral therapy is currently being evaluated. Patients with symptomatic HIV infection, AIDS Related Complex (ARC) and AIDS require specialist management of the opportunistic infections and neoplasms which they develop.

SYSTEMIC STD AND PREGNANCY

For many years, women attending antenatal clinics have been screened for syphilis and often hepatitis B infection, on serum samples obtained at their booking visit. There is now an increasing trend for HIV antibody testing to be offered as well. However, it is generally accepted that this must be accompanied by a more detailed and informative pretest counselling service than previously available. Indeed, much of the discussion about HIV antibody testing is leading to a reappraisal of the suitability of using pregnancy as a time to carry out opportunistic screening of women.

Ideally, the time to diagnose asymptomatic infections, which might be transmitted vertically, is prior to the pregnancy, as part of comprehensive preconceptual care. But, even if this service was widely available and infected women were identified prior to conception, would any therapy alter the pregnancy outcome?

Syphilis

Vertical transmission via the placenta is almost inevitable if the mother is suffering from secondary syphilis and is reasonably likely if she has a primary chancre, but becomes more unlikely with increasing duration of latent disease. In 30% of women with untreated early syphilis, the pregnancy will end in a second trimester spontaneous abortion or still-birth. If a live infant results, it may rarely be born showing signs of early congenital syphilis, or more usually be born well, developing signs within the first few weeks, months or even years of life. With successive pregnancies, the outcome tends to improve.

Adequate treatment of maternal syphilis prior to a pregnancy will prevent any transmission to the fetus or infant. It should be remembered that infection of the mother may also occur during pregnancy and therefore screening at 14–16 weeks' gestation will not prevent all cases of congenital infection. Furthermore, if reinfection is considered a possibility during a pregnancy, then retreatment is essential.

Hepatitis B

Infection of a pregnant woman carries a mortality of 1.8% and a 20% increase in preterm delivery, although there is no specific association with congenital abnormalities. These figures relate to Europe and North America, but in India and the Far East, fulminant hepatitis is more common with a reported maternal mortality of 72% for cases of third trimester infection. The reason for this geographical variation is thought to include ethnic differences in host immunity. A geographical difference also exists in the risk of vertical transmission by a mother who is a chronic carrier of hepatitis B surface antigen (HBsAg) throughout her pregnancy. This varies from a 7% risk of vertical transmission in Greece, compared to 73% in Japan. These differences seem to be directly related to the titre of HBsAg and also the presence of e antigen in maternal serum.

For infections acquired during pregnancy, the risk of vertical transmission to the fetus is determined by the gestational age at the time of maternal infection. A third trimester infection carries a 66% risk of transmission, compared to less than 10% if the virus is acquired earlier.

There is no evidence that any therapy given during pregnancy alters the risk of transmission or the maternal or perinatal morbidity. However, to prevent the risk of neonatal transmission, infants born of HBsAg positive mothers should receive hepatitis B immunoglobulin and a dose of hepatitis B vaccine, at separate sites, within a few hours of birth.

HIV infection

Early reports that pregnancy in an HIV infected woman resulted in an increased rate of progression to AIDS have not been substantiated. The immunological changes seen in uninfected women seem to be replicated (with postnatal recovery) in HIV infected women, but at a lower absolute level.

Pregnancy outcome does not appear to be affected by HIV infection when compared to that of comparable HIV seronegative women from similar social groups (e.g. intravenous drug users in poor housing conditions). A rare embryopathy has been described, but the true incidence of this complication has yet to be confirmed.

Vertical transmission appears to occur in 30–40% of infants delivered to HIV infected women. It has been suggested that this risk of transmission may be highest during periods of significant HIV p24 antigenaemia, especially during the seroconversion illness and in patients with ARC and AIDS. It is uncertain at which stage of pregnancy or delivery the transmission of HIV to the fetus usually occurs. Examination of aborted material has revealed transplacental transmission as early as 16 weeks' gestation.

The diagnosis of HIV infection in children is difficult due to the problem of passive acquisition of maternal HIV antibodies. The persistence of HIV antibody after 15 months is thought to indicate infection, but new techniques for viral detection may make earlier diagnosis possible.

The detection of HIV in breast milk has resulted in advice that infants born to HIV antibody positive mothers should not be breast-fed, nor should these mothers contribute to milk banks.

The risk of transmission of HIV to obstetric and midwifery staff has been a source of much discussion. The role of antenatal screening of pregnant women for HIV infection is currently being debated, as to whether it is ethical, should be voluntary or compulsory and how to provide adequate pre- and post-test counselling. The current advice to staff in obstetric and gynaecological units is to treat all women with similar careful precautions. Indeed, the overall risk of transmission of HIV from patients to healthcare workers seems to be low, at around 0.4% after penetrating needlestick injuries involving HIV infected blood. However, as with many problems associated with HIV infection, only further studies will reveal whether current management strategies are sufficient.

SUMMARY

The historical importance of syphilis as 'the great mimic' of any other condition is being superseded by the vast range of symptoms and signs associated with HIV infection. Currently 8% of cases of HIV infection in the UK have occurred in women and this proportion is increasing. The majority of these women are intravenous drug users, but one-third of cases have been infected by heterosexual contact. With increasing numbers of women with HIV infection, the importance of a high level of clinical awareness and surveillance for this condition is essential.

37. Family planning

C. Watson

Expectations of the examiners

The candidate will be expected to have the following theoretical knowledge:

1. The factors influencing motivation for contraception and emotional/psychological factors related to fertility control.
2. The acceptability, effectiveness and safety of all available methods of contraception (including sterilization) with their advantages/disadvantages and risks/benefits.
3. How to provide counselling/advice to the couple choosing any contraceptive method and how to manage associated complications (including resuscitation if required at IUCD insertion).
4. The organization of family planning services.

MOTIVATION FOR CONTRACEPTION

The following factors are known to be influential in determining whether a couple will seek contraception:

1. The personal/cultural ideal family size
2. The sex of the existing children in the family
3. Religious beliefs
4. Socioeconomic conditions
5. Expected dependency or assistance from children
6. Opportunities and education for women
7. The stage in family building
8. Age and marital status
9. The stability of the male/female relationship
10. The perceived risk of pregnancy
11. The availability of information about contraceptive services
12. Expectations about the confidentiality of services.

ACCEPTABILITY OF CONTRACEPTIVE METHODS

Even when a couple are motivated to use contraception, they may find their choice of method difficult and may finally opt for a method which is seen simply as the least of several evils. They will be influenced by the following factors:

1. Effectiveness of the method
2. Perceived safety of the method
3. Whether the method is used by the man or the woman
4. Convenience and simplicity in use
5. Whether action is required at the time of coitus
6. Freedom from forethought
7. Whether the method is well-known or novel
8. Whether or not the method has religious approval
9. Availability of the method.

CONTRACEPTIVE CHOICE

In order to cater for as many needs and preferences as possible it is important that couples are free to choose their source of advice and their method of contraception. Confidentiality may be of particular importance to some groups, e.g. young people. The role of the professional is to give information and after history/examination to advise the individual/couple of any factors which might influence the effectiveness or safety of the method(s) they may be contemplating. The final choice should be with the individual/couple, and is likely to be most successful when the couple are in agreement.

Commonly, a couple will opt to use more than one method during their reproductive life, changing their method to suit changing circumstances, e.g.:

1. First using the combined pill to *delay* onset of childbearing
2. Then using an IUCD to *space* their children
3. Finally using sterilization when the family is *complete*.

EFFECTIVENESS

Definitions

Theoretical effectiveness is defined as what might be achieved under 'ideal' circumstances but in practice is never achieved.

User-effectiveness is defined as that actually achieved in practice.

Method-failure is defined as failure inherent to the method itself.

User-failure is defined as failure due to using a method inadequately or not at all.

Some methods of contraception are particularly vulnerable to 'user-failure', e.g. oral contraceptives and condoms, while others are almost entirely vulnerable to 'method-failure', e.g. IUCDs and sterilization.

Measurements of effectiveness

Pearl index

This method takes into account the length of time the woman has been exposed to the risk of pregnancy. It is expressed in terms of a rate per 100 woman-years (HWY) and is calculated as follows:

$$\text{Failure rate per HWY} = \frac{\text{Total no. of pregnancies} \times 1200}{\text{Total months of use for all those using method}}$$

Life-table analysis

This method takes into account the changing probability of pregnancy over a period of time and is therefore more accurate. Calculations are expressed in terms of a rate per 100 women after 'n' months or years of use.

The effectiveness of any method varies in practice with differences due to personal, social and cultural factors in the user, the provider, and the user–provider relationship. When user-failure is important, failure rates are highest in couples who are young or inexperienced. Fertility diminishes with age, particularly sharply in women after the age of 35 with consequent lowering of failure rates.

For the purposes of counselling patients, methods may be usefully classified into three groups according to the 'best results that can be obtained in practice'.

1. Very highly effective (failures less than 1 per HWY)
   a. Sterilization (male or female)
   b. Combined oestrogen/progestogen pills (COC)
   c. Depot progestogen injections.
2. Highly effective (failures 2–3 per HWY)
   a. Progestogen-only pills (POP)
   b. Intrauterine contraceptive devices (IUCDs)
   c. Diaphragm/cap with spermicide
   d. Condom with spermicide
   e. Periodic abstinence (symptothermal method).
3. Moderately effective (failures may exceed 10 per HWY)
   a. Spermicide alone
   b. Contraceptive sponge
   c. Periodic abstinence (calendar method)
   d. Coitus interruptus
   e. Home-made barriers and spermicides.

SAFETY

Contraceptive safety should be assessed in comparison with the morbidity and mortality associated with pregnancy. Where maternal mortality and morbidity are high, e.g. Latin America and Africa, the relative safety of contraceptive methods is very great. In developed countries the mortality associated with different contraceptive methods, their known failure rates, and the mortality associated with pregnancy can be used to compute relative risks for sexually active women. From such studies it would appear that:

1. For women under 30 who do not smoke, mortality risks without contraception are of the order of 1–2 deaths per 100 000 women per year compared with 5–7 deaths per 100 000 from unregulated fertility.
2. Women over the age of 35 who smoke and take the COC have an increased mortality which at least equals that associated with pregnancy.
3. For all other methods over the age of 30, overall mortality in contracepting women remains well below the mortality associated with pregnancy in non-contracepting women.
4. At all ages, the lowest level of overall mortality is achieved by using barrier methods of contraception with recourse to first trimester abortion in cases of failure.

STERILIZATION

Popularity

The General Household Survey (1983) revealed that 22% of couples aged 18–44 in England and Wales relied on sterilization as their method of contraception. Male and female methods were equally used.

Methods

Bilateral vasectomy in the male and tubal procedures performed at laparoscopy or minilaparotomy in the female are the preferred methods. Clips or rings are now used in preference to diathermy for female sterilization. Interval sterilization has a better prognosis than sterilization carried out in association with pregnancy.

Advantages

1. Very highly effective.
2. Needs no continuing motivation.
3. One-time procedure with no ongoing costs.
4. Safe: side-effects and health hazards are rare.

Disadvantages

1. Regret is possible. Reversal is expensive and cannot be guaranteed.

Table 37.1   Implications of the male and female sterilization options.

	Male	Female
Immediacy	Not immediately effective	Immediately effective
Failure	Less than 0.5% in first year	Less than 0.5% in first year
Mortality	1 in 100 000 (mostly under LA)	1 in 10 000 (mostly under GA)
Morbidity		
Early	Below 5% (bleeding, infection)	Below 5% (bleeding, infection, trauma)
Late	Sperm granuloma	Ectopic pregnancy
Reversibility	Chances dependent on extent of original procedure	
Availability	Marked regional/district variations	

2. Needs surgeon/special equipment, i.e. relatively large capital outlay which tends to restrict availability.

Importance of counselling the couple

From the medicolegal point of view it is important to stress both the irreversibility of the procedure and the very small failure rate. Alternative contraception should be discussed as well as the implications of the male and female sterilization options (Table 37.1).

HORMONAL CONTRACEPTION

Mechanism of action

The sex steroids (oestrogens and progestogens) used in available hormonal contraceptive preparations have the following actions:

1. Hypothalamus and pituitary—inhibition of CnRH FSH and LH via 'feedback' system.
2. Ovary—consequent inhibition of follicular activity, ovulation and luteal function.
3. Endometrium—inadequate secretory phase prejudices implantation.
4. Cervical mucus—progestogens render it resistant to sperm penetration.
5. Fallopian tubes—impaired function interferes with sperm/ovum transport.

Note: These actions are dose-dependent and vary from one woman to another.

COMBINED OESTROGEN-PROGESTOGEN PILLS (COC)

Popularity

Currently used by 60 million women worldwide, this method is the most popular in the UK. Since first marketed in the early 60s, the dose of oestrogen and then the dose of progestogen has been greatly reduced with a current trend to introduce newer progestogens which interfere less with lipid profiles.

N.B. ↑ rate DVT/PE cf old ones.

Advantages

1. Contraceptive
   a. Very highly effective
   b. Convenient—no action required at time of coitus
   c. Reversible—does not cause subsequent infertility.
2. Non-contraceptive benefits
   a. Improvement in the menstrual cycle:
      i. Reduced blood loss—less iron deficiency anaemia
      ii. Reduced dysmenorrhoea
      iii. Reduced premenstrual problems
      iv. Prevention of 'mittelschmerz' (ovulation pain/bleeding)
      v. Increased regularity of bleeding (withdrawal bleeds)
      vi. Ability to manipulate the cycle, e.g. tri-cycle regime.
   b. Reduction in gynaecological disease and need for surgery
      i. Reduction in benign breast tumours
      ii. Reduction in ovarian cysts, fibroids, endometriosis
      iii. Reduction in pelvic inflammatory disease, therefore
      iv. Reduction in tubal infertility and ectopic pregnancy
      v. Reduction in ovarian and endometrial cancers (both duration of use and ex-use effects).
   c. Other possible or minor benefits
      i. Reduction in seborrhoeic conditions
      ii. Reduction in thyroid disease, peptic ulcer and rheumatoid arthritis.

Disadvantages

1. Requires continuous motivation to take the pill correctly.
2. Requires medical supervision.
3. Not immediately effective unless started on first day of cycle.
4. Minor side-effects may be experienced, especially in the early months of use, e.g. nausea, breast discomfort, weight gain, headache (unusual with modern low-dose pills) or 'break-through bleeding'.
5. For a minority of women there may be serious health hazards and so screening for contraindications should take place before prescribing.

Cardiovascular disease

An observed increase in venous thromboembolic disease has been attributed to oestrogen-induced changes in clotting factors. An observed increase in arterial disease (ischaemic heart disease and cerebrovascular disease) has been attributed to oestrogen-induced changes in clotting factors plus progestogen-induced changes in serum lipids (mainly HDL reduction). Oestrogens may also raise angiotensin II and thereby contribute to the development of hypertension in some women. Epidemiological studies have demonstrated a lowering of risks with lower dose pills and excess mortality and morbidity from cardiovascular disease appears to be confined almost completely to women over the age of 35 who smoke.

Neoplasia

Carcinoma of the breast. There is no consistent evidence linking an overall excess incidence of breast cancer with COC use. Evidence is conflicting on a possible increase in breast cancer presenting in younger women after early COC use. Data from women on low-dose pills is still insufficient.

Carcinoma of the cervix. There is some evidence of an association between COC use and an increased risk of CIN/invasive cancer but a causal relationship is not established due to lack of information about confounding factors, e.g. sexual behaviour.

Liver tumours. Benign and malignant tumours may be increased by long-term use of high-dose pills but are extremely rare.

Contraindications to COC use

Absolute (but some not permanent)

1. Hormone-dependent tumours—breast, endometrial, trophoblastic.
2. Cardiovascular disease
   a. Venous—thromboembolism or thrombophlebitis
   b. Arterial—ischaemic heart disease, cerebrovascular disease, peripheral vascular disease, Raynaud's disease
   c. Valvular heart disease—with risk of embolization or pulmonary hypertension
   d. Migraine—commencing on COC or focal
   e. Increased clotting tendency—immobility, homozygous sickle cell disease, elective surgery and during treatment of varicose veins (sclerosant therapy or surgery).
3. Impaired liver or renal function including active hepatitis, cholestatic jaundice of pregnancy, certain rare inherited disorders, e.g. Dubin–Johnson and Rotor's syndromes.
4. Serious conditions known to have been made worse by previous pregnancy or sex steroids, e.g. otosclerosis, chorea, porphyria.

Relative (more than one in combination may be a very strong contraindication)

1. Age over 35 years
2. Current smoker
3. Hypertension
4. Hyperlipidaemia
5. Diabetes
6. Obesity
7. Family history of premature cardiovascular disease
8. Lactation
9. Puerperal psychosis/severe mood disorder
10. Sickle cell trait
11. Migraine (not as above)
12. Asthma
13. Epilepsy
14. Some diseases may be made worse by COC effect on immune mechanisms, e.g. Crohn's disease
15. Hyperprolactinaemia.

Note: There is no evidence that COC use prejudices future fertility in the long term but women with a history of oligomenorrhoea require pre-treatment information on this point and women with amenorrhoea in excess of six months require investigation prior to treatment.

Prescribing principles

Choose

1. Low oestrogen dose (20–35 micrograms ethinyl oestradiol)
2. Low progestogen dose: first choice: 500 micrograms norethisterone or 150 micrograms levonorgestrel
3. Avoid pro-drugs (only pharmacologically active as metabolites)
4. Monophasic regime which is simple for the patient
5. Low cost preparation.

Note: Newer progestogens (desogestrel and gestodene) have been developed to reduce the depressant effect on HDL cholesterol. Claims for the superiority of these more expensive preparations can only be substantiated by long-term epidemiological studies and at present must remain speculative. Use of these COCs and the more expensive and complicated phased preparations may be justified in women with relative contra-indications or in the management of side-effects. *Only use if intolerant of old ones and no ↑ risk DVT / PE.*

Practical prescribing

1. The lowest dose monophasic preparation should be prescribed first and the patient warned to expect spotting or break-through bleeding for up

to the fourth month of use. If cycle control is not attained by then, the dose of progestogen may be increased. (An increase in oestrogen is not usually desirable.)

2. The simplest regime is to advise the patient to take her first ever pill on the first day of menstrual bleeding and to continue with 21 consecutive pills (one per day) followed by a 7-day break. The COC is then immediately effective, and a regular 28-day 'cycle' is the norm. The COC may be commenced immediately after therapeutic abortion or 3–4 weeks after childbirth.

3. Contraceptive efficacy may be lost if pills are forgotten (more than 12 hours late), malabsorbed, or subjected to drug interaction. An alternative contraceptive method should be advised during the lapse and for seven days after reinstitution of effective COC use, but when an enzyme-inducing drug is used, contraceptive efficacy may not be regained until eight weeks after cessation of therapy. If the seven days extends into the 'pill-free' week, two packs of 21 pills should be taken consecutively without a break.

4. The most important drug interactions which may affect contraceptive efficacy are:
   a. Broad-spectrum antibiotics which may impair oestrogen reabsorption in the enterohepatic circulation (affects COC only)
   b. Enzyme-inducing drugs (rifampicin, griseofulvin, anticonvulsants) which interfere with oestrogen and progestogen metabolism in the liver (affects COC and POP). Patients wishing to use the COC and enzyme-inducers should be prescribed a COC with a high dose of oestrogen (50 micrograms) and progestogen.

5. COCs should be stopped six weeks in advance of elective surgery if possible to allow clotting factors to normalize.

6. All patients need careful teaching about how to take the COC and careful counselling about what to expect. This information should also be given in writing. Family Planning Information Service (FPIS) free leaflets are available for this purpose.

PROGESTOGEN-ONLY PILLS (POP)

Mechanisms of action

Their effects on ovulation, endometrium and tubal function are variable, hence there is difficulty in predicting menstrual patterns. They are more effective if taken regularly about 4–6 hours before the likely time of intercourse to maximize the effect on cervical mucus.

Advantages

1. No significant metabolic effects and they can therefore be used in lactating mothers, older women, diabetics, etc.

2. Can be used when oestrogens are contraindicated.
3. Continuous daily regime may be simpler for patient to remember.

Disadvantages

1. As for disadvantages 1–3 of combined oestrogen/progestogen pills
2. Less effective than COCs. The failure rate is age-related (0–4%)
3. Possible menstrual irregularity (spotting, short cycles or amenorrhoea) which may prove unacceptable to the patient
4. The *relative risk* of ectopic pregnancy is increased
5. Increased risk of developing functional ovarian cysts due to partial suppression of follicular development—may cause diagnostic confusion with suspected ectopic pregnancy.

Contraindications to POP use

1. Hormone-dependent tumours (unless agreed with oncologist)
2. A past history of ectopic pregnancy is a relative contraindication as methods which consistently prevent ovulation offer more protection against a recurrence.

Prescribing principles

There is no convincing evidence that any preparation is superior to another, therefore the cheapest should be prescribed.

Practical prescribing

1. Start the first pill on the first day of menstrual bleeding and continue with one pill daily at the same time of day. After pregnancy the POP may be started immediately (regardless of gestation).
2. Contraceptive efficacy may be lost if pills are forgotten (more than 3 hours late), malabsorbed or subjected to drug interaction from enzyme-inducing drugs which will have an effect for up to eight weeks from discontinuation. An alternative contraceptive method should be used during the period at risk and for ~~48 hours~~ *7 days* thereafter.
3. Instruction and counselling of the patient should be reinforced by written information (FPIS leaflets).

DEPOT PROGESTOGEN INJECTIONS

Mechanisms of action

The dose of progestogen is sufficiently large to inhibit ovulation fairly consistently. The endometrium tends to become atrophic with no secretory activity, and cervical mucus thickens.

Advantages

1. Very highly effective, and immediately if given in first five days of the cycle. No user-failure between injections
2. Convenient, requiring no continuous motivation or action at time of coitus
3. Safe—no mortality reported
4. Reversible—does not cause permanent infertility
5. Private—can be used unknown to uncooperative male partner
6. Lactation not suppressed—may be enhanced
7. Can be used when oestrogens contraindicated
8. Erythropoiesis stimulated. Reduces crises in homozygous sickle cell disease
9. Probable reduction in menstrual disorders and gynaecological disease as for COC (with exception of irregular bleeding but amenorrhoea usually supervenes with continuing use).

Disadvantages

1. Cannot 'stop' in an emergency
2. Some women dislike injections
3. Requires medical supervision
4. May be some delay in return of fertility after use (up to 2 years but usually about 6 months)
5. Bleeding irregularities may be unacceptable to the patient
6. Weight gain—affects some patients
7. Measurable metabolic effects on glucose tolerance (reduced) and HDL cholesterol (reduced) but significance unknown
8. Theoretical risk of fetal masculinization if norethisterone oenanthate given in pregnancy
9. May cause galactorrhoea.

Contraindications

1. Pregnancy—present or desired in near future
2. Anxiety about possible menstrual disturbance
3. Best avoided in early postpartum period (increases risk of heavy bleeding) and in breast-feeding mothers of premature infants (as excreted in small quantities in breast milk).

Practical prescribing

Depo-Provera (DMPA—medroxyprogesterone acetate) and Noristerat (NET OEN—norethisterone oenanthate) are both marketed in the UK and may be offered to patients after information and counselling. Manufacturer's information leaflets and audiotapes are available for Depo-Provera in English and a number of ethnic minority languages. Noristerat has a product licence for short-term use as a contraceptive. The usual doses are Depo-Provera 150 mg 12-weekly or Noristerat 200 mg 8-weekly. Both should be given by deep intramuscular injection into the gluteal muscle.

Patients should be screened initially and at follow-up as for the COC and POP (BP, weight, breast and pelvic exam plus cervical smear). Excessive bleeding (defined as more than 7 days out of 21) should be actively managed after excluding other causes of bleeding.

Within one month of the injection, a small dose of oestrogen may be beneficial (e.g. ethinyl oestradiol 10 µg daily for 10 days). Bleeding in the latter half of the injection interval should be managed by an additional dose e.g. Depo-Provera 50 mg i.m. or by rescheduling the next injection to an earlier date.

INTRAUTERINE CONTRACEPTIVE DEVICES (IUCD)

Popularity

Worldwide popularity is equal to that of oral contraceptives. An estimated 60 million women are current users of IUCDs.

Mechanisms of action

Alteration/inhibition of sperm migration, fertilization and ovum transport, plus production of a sterile inflammatory response in the endometrium which inhibits implantation of the blastocyst. It may therefore be used as a postcoital method and should not be removed from the uterus within seven days of coitus if pregnancy is not desired.

Advantages

1. Safe—mortality is very rare and there are no metabolic effects
2. Highly effective and effective immediately or postcoitally
3. Continuation rates high as the method proves acceptable to the majority of women who choose it
4. Reversible
5. Requires no sustained motivation or action at time of coitus
6. Can provide long-term contraception cheaply.

Disadvantages

1. Need specially trained personnel to fit and give follow-up care
2. Possible complications at time of insertion of the device include pain, bleeding, vagal inhibition and perforation of the uterus

3. Later complications may include pregnancy (including an increased relative risk of ectopic pregnancy), pain, bleeding, expulsion, displacement, infection or problems with the threads (lost threads or male dyspareunia).

Contraindications to IUCD use

Absolute

1. Pregnancy
2. Acute or chronic pelvic infection
3. Certain congenital abnormalities of the uterus
4. Large fibroids which distort the uterine cavity
5. Wilson's disease or Copper allergy.

Relative

1. Menorrhagia
2. Malignant disease of the genital tract
3. Fixed retroversion of the uterus
4. Past history of ectopic pregnancy or pelvic inflammatory disease
5. Nulliparity
6. Congenital or rheumatic heart disease (may require antibiotic cover for insertion)
7. Diabetes mellitus
8. Systemic steroid or immunosuppressive therapy.

Prevention and management of complications

Potential patients should be carefully screened for contraindications by history, examination and investigation if necessary.

Insertion of the device should be carried out in a calm, relaxed manner with due attention to aseptic technique and analgesia for the patient if necessary. Vagal inhibition resulting in bradycardia and a fall in blood pressure should be managed by placing the patient in the semiprone (recovery) position with the head tilted downwards 10–15°. An airway should be inserted if there is any loss of consciousness and persistent bradycardia may be treated by i.v. atropine 0.6 mg.

The device may have to be removed if menstrual pain and bleeding are unacceptable. Intermenstrual pain/bleeding may be due to infection or partial expulsion/displacement of the device. Suspected infection should be treated promptly in a department of genitourinary medicine with follow-up of the partner.

Perforation may be suspected when threads are absent and may be investigated by ultrasound. If confirmed, laparoscopic removal of the device should be arranged without delay. If pregnancy occurs with the device in situ, the patient should be advised to have the device removed immediately while the threads are accessible. Previous expulsion is not a contraindication to the insertion of another device.

Practical prescribing

The devices available in the UK are:

1. Ortho Gyne-T, Ortho Gyne-T 380 Slimline
2. Multiload Cu 250 (short and standard), Multiload Cu 375
3. Nova T/Novagard.

The choice of device may be made on the basis of uterine size and tightness of the cervix as determined by sounding the uterus, but the choice of device is probably less important than the selection of the patient and the skill of the operator. IUCDs may be fitted at any time in the menstrual cycle if contraception has been used effectively. After delivery it is customary to wait until six weeks postpartum for insertion but devices may be fitted at the time of delivery if appropriate and also at the time of termination of pregnancy.

Despite the varying recommendations of the manufacturers it is likely that all devices can be left in utero for five years without loss of efficacy. The Ortho Gyne-T 380 Slimline does not require periodic replacement.

BARRIER METHODS OF CONTRACEPTION

Popularity

There has been renewed interest in barrier contraceptives in response to concern about HIV infection. Theory and clinical experience suggest that maximum contraceptive efficacy can only be obtained by using a barrier and spermicide together. The commonly used spermicide, Nonoxynol-9 has been shown to be active against HIV virus in vitro.

Advantages

1. Protection from sexually transmitted infection
2. Protection from carcinoma of the cervix
3. Instantly effective (after initial learning)
4. No systemic side-effects
5. Caps do not interfere with the sensation of either partner (although condoms are reputed to do so)
6. Available from non-medical sources.

Disadvantages

1. Need trained personnel to fit cap initially and check periodically
2. Require continuous motivation and supplies
3. Action required at time of coitus (for condom use)
4. 'User-failure' can be high, e. g. the young/inexperienced
5. Couples may find barrier methods messy or distasteful
6. Small increase in cystitis/vaginal infections in cap users.

Practical prescribing

CAP

There are two types of cap:

1. Diaphragm (flat-spring, coil-spring and arcing types). These can be successful when the pelvic floor has good muscle tone.
2. Suction cap (cervical, vault and vimule types). These can be used when there is prolapse of the vaginal walls.

The patient should be fitted with a suitable cap and then taught how to remove and reinsert the device several times under supervision before she relies on the method. She should also be instructed in the correct use of spermicide and be given written instructions on the use of the method (see FPIS leaflet).

Periodic checks of the fitting and correct placement of the cap should take place during use.

CONDOMS

These may be dispensed free of charge in hospitals and community health family planning clinics. They vary in shape, thickness, and lubrication. They may have features, e.g. texture or colour, designed to enhance their attractiveness to the user. Some brands now have a spermicide incorporated in the lubricant. There is a British standard for condoms and those without the 'kitemark' should not be used.

Clients should be given detailed instructions in the use of condoms and should also be made aware of the availability of postcoital contraceptive methods. (See FPIS leaflets.)

SPERMICIDES

These are available as tubed creams, jellies or pastes, aerosol foam, soluble pessaries, foaming tablets, and water-soluble plastic film. High failure rates would be expected if they are used without a barrier.

Note: Oil-based spermicides or other products should not be used with caps/condoms as they can damage the tensile strength of the rubber.

SPONGES

Disposable contraceptive sponges, impregnated with the spermicide Nonoxynol-9 are marketed in the UK but are not available on prescription. They are relatively expensive and ineffective.

PERIODIC ABSTINENCE

This method is also referred to as natural family planning, the rhythm method or the safe period. It is based on the principle of avoidance of coitus during the 'fertile days' of a woman's menstrual cycle but in practice this is difficult to determine because:

1. Sperm may survive in the female genital tract for up to seven days postcoitus
2. Ovulation cannot be predicted accurately seven days in advance.

High effectiveness can therefore only be achieved by restricting coitus to the postovulatory phase of the cycle after the ovum is presumed to be incapable of being fertilized.

The most accurate way of determining the 'infertile' days is to use various methods in combination—the 'symptothermal' method:

1. Observation from a menstrual calendar of the longest cycle length and calculation of the last fertile day by subtracting 10.
2. Observation of basal body temperature and reckoning on the infertile phase beginning on the third morning of elevated temperature readings following midcycle release of the ovum.
3. Observations of cervical elevation and softening at the time of ovulation; ovulatory pain, bleeding or breast discomfort; and serial observations of cervical mucus. The infertile phase is reckoned to begin on the fourth evening after peak mucus production.

Advantages

1. Free of any known physical side-effects
2. May be acceptable to couples whose religion or culture debars them from other methods
3. Always available and cheap (after teaching)
4. The knowledge gained by couples practising the method may also assist them when planning conception.

Disadvantages

1. High user-failure rates which vary between six and 25 pregnancies per HWY
2. The infertile period may be difficult to identify, e.g. during fever

3. The couple have to accept considerable limitations on the days available for coitus. Sustained motivation and cooperation are essential to success.

Practical prescribing

Temperature charts and fertility thermometers are available on prescription in the UK. The couple should be counselled and taught effectively and offered on-going support. A FPIS leaflet is available.

POSTCOITAL CONTRACEPTION

A request for this emergency method of contraception should lead to a review of the couple's on-going contraceptive strategy. In order that the method can be used at all, the population needs to be educated about its existence and availability. The method should be accessible on every day of the week.

There are two methods:

1. *Hormonal.* The most popular regime is the one recommended by Yuzpe: Ovran 50 (levonorgestrel 250 micrograms plus ethinyloestradiol 50 micrograms) two tablets stat followed by two tablets 12 hours later. This must be instituted within 72 hours of unprotected coitus. Prior exposure to conception in the current cycle outside the 72-hour period is a contraindication. The next menstrual period may occur on schedule, early or late. Slight nausea may affect about 30% of takers. Ectopic pregnancy is a theoretical increased risk and a past history of ectopic pregnancy may be a relative contraindication. The overall failure rate is approximately 2%. ~5% dep. upon time in cycle.
2. *IUCD insertion.* This is effective if fitted within five days of exposure to unprotected coitus (without prior exposure earlier in the cycle). Nulliparity and rape are relative contraindications because of the greater susceptibility to sexually transmitted infection. A past history of ectopic pregnancy is a strong contraindication. The method is virtually 100% effective and may be retained by the women as her on-going method or removed with the next period if so desired.

ORGANIZATION OF FAMILY PLANNING SERVICES

Family planning services in the UK were mainly provided by the Family Planning Association until they were transferred to the National Health Service with reorganization in 1974. The intention was that all who needed advice and help with family planning (regardless of sex or marital status) should be able to choose a free service from the following sources (DHSS Circular HSC(1S) 32 May 1974):

1. Community health services

2. Hospital services
3. Family practitioner services.

These services should be seen as complementary to each other and liaison should be encouraged.

COMMUNITY HEALTH SERVICES

Family planning advice and supplies may be delivered by:

1. Community midwives and health visitors
2. Community family planning clinics
3. Special youth advisory centres
4. Domiciliary family planning services.

HOSPITAL SERVICES

Family planning advice and supplies may be delivered by:

1. Hospital midwives working in antenatal/postnatal clinics and parent-craft classes
2. Hospital outpatient family planning clinics
3. Hospital family planning 'visitors' who see patients in postnatal and postabortion wards
4. Hospital gynaecology clinics especially TOP request clinics
5. Hospital staff in any department may find it appropriate to advise or refer patients as part of their regular clinical care.

FAMILY PRACTITIONER SERVICES

General practitioners may choose to provide family planning services within normal surgery hours and/or in special 'sessions'.

38. Psychosexual counselling

C. Watson

Expectations of the examiners

The candidate will be expected to have an understanding of the principles involved in counselling patients with psychosexual problems.

Definition

Human sexuality involves gender identity, sexual object choice, sexual drive and sexual function (behaviour). Individuals display wide variations in these parameters and therefore it is a general principle to assert that it is the client who decides whether any particular state is a 'problem'. Doctors should be sensitive to this issue and should not make assumptions about their patient's wishes.

Examples of these problems are:

1. Problem of gender identity—transsexualism
2. Problem of sexual object choice—fetishism
3. Problem of sexual drive—hypogonadism
4. Problem of sexual function—vaginismus.

Interesting facts

The true incidence of any aspect of human sexuality is not known but complaints about sexual problems are common and most relate to sexual dysfunction, i.e. problems of sexual function or interest. There is ample evidence nonetheless, that many patients find it difficult to ask for professional help in this area and that of those who do, the sexual dysfunction may be associated with other more fundamental problems in the relationship or the personality. It is also likely that many patients experience sexual dysfunction but do not regard it as a problem.

Pathophysiology

Sexual dysfunctions which impede or prevent a couple from having or enjoying sexual intercourse include the conditions listed in Table 38.1.

Table 38.1 Sexual dysfunctions.

Disorders	In the woman	In the man
Initiation	Lack of interest	Lack of interest
Sexual arousal	Failure of lubrication and swelling response	Erectile impotence
Penetration	Vaginismus	,, ,,
	Dyspareunia	Dyspareunia
Orgasm	Failure of orgasm	Premature ejaculation
		Retarded ejaculation

Problems in one partner almost always affect the other and an individual or couple may have more than one coexisting difficulty. For example, it is common to find premature ejaculation in the male partner accompanied by orgasmic dysfunction in the female partner. Sexual dysfunctions may also be classified according to whether they are primary or secondary to a period of normal function.

Aetiology

Psychological factors always play a part in sexual dysfunction even when physical factors are mainly responsible. Counselling the individual or couple is therefore an important element of management.

Physical causes of sexual dysfunction

Illness. Any physical or mental illness may be expected to interfere with sexual life. Chronic illness, stress, fatigue and depression may be associated with loss of sexual interest. Vascular disease and neuropathy, e.g. in diabetics, may prevent erection. Endocrine disorders which reduce free testosterone may be associated with lack of sexual drive. It is common for women to experience a loss of sexual interest after childbirth which may be attributed to a complex interaction of stressful life-events, fatigue, hormonal changes (particularly in the lactating mother) and possible dyspareunia from an episiotomy scar.

Age. Although many individuals/couples enjoy sexual expression well into old age, most will have to adjust to changes in their sexual responsiveness as they become older. Erectile impotence is a common complaint in men over 50 which may simply reflect a general reduction in sexual responsiveness and the need for more tactile stimulation but organic factors (as yet imperfectly understood) may also be important.

Drugs. Many drugs (both therapeutic and recreational) can affect sexual functioning. Alcohol probably inhibits sexual response through central nervous system effects.

Psychological causes of sexual dysfunction

Immediate causes

Learning difficulties. Sexual ignorance continues to play a small part in sexual problems. Unrealistic expectations may also contribute to sexual dissatisfaction (for example if 'vaginal orgasm' is believed to be the 'norm' for women). Couples sometimes do not relate their socioeconomic difficulties, e.g. living virtually without privacy, to the sexual problems they are experiencing.

Sexual anxiety. Sexual anxiety can prevent the physiological changes of sexual arousal and contribute to premature ejaculation in the man. Fear of failure makes a major contribution to erectile impotence in men who may feel that they are expected to 'perform'. Other men who experience premature ejaculation may have an excessive need to please their partner and may be so overconcerned about this that they are unable to focus on their own sexual pleasure.

Lack of communication between the sexual partners. Some couples find it difficult to talk about sexual matters and may therefore give less pleasure to each other than they could if they knew more about each other's preferences. Feelings of rejection and guilt may develop due to lack of understanding and can cause unnecessary distress.

Underlying causes

Relationship difficulties between the partners. Lack of commitment, lack of trust and disappointment in the partner may be associated with sexual problems which are unlikely to improve unless the basic relationship difficulties can be resolved.

Personal difficulties. Each partner may have difficulties which may relate to their upbringing, past experience and attitudes towards sexuality. They may experience conflict with the idea that sexual behaviour should be pleasurable and feel consequent guilt and shame. Negative sexual experiences such as childhood sexual abuse or rape may contribute to these difficulties.

Assessment

As most people still find it difficult to present their sexual problems, the attitude of the professional to whom they first unburden themselves is extremely important.

The attitude of the doctor is probably more important than any specific knowledge or skill in treating sexual problems. Many individuals/couples will be helped at a 'primary' level by the following features in the therapist:

1. Listening skills and the use of open-ended questions
2. Genuine concern about the patient
3. Lack of embarassment—being at ease with sexual matters

4. A non-judgmental attitude and avoidance of 'standard-setting'
5. Avoidance of medical jargon and use of ordinary language.

As the problem unfolds it may become apparent that 'secondary' or specialist help is needed but it is important not to refer the patient on too quickly in case they may feel rejected and unable to contemplate the process of unburdening themselves a second time to another professional.

Because of the difficulties felt by patients, sexual problems may not be overtly expressed but may present covertly with another complaint which may well relate to the sexual organs, their function or contraception. Doctors working in gynaecological situations need to be alert to complaints which may serve as a 'ticket of entry' to the 'real problem' which is a sexual one. Common presentations include complaints of dyspareunia, discharge, pelvic pain, or 'side-effects' from the contraceptive pill. These complaints will normally require a careful history, examination and possible investigation before it can be agreed that they have their origin in psychological distress. There is also the possibility that both a physical and psychological problem may coexist or that a physical problem may be the cause of sexual dysfunction, e.g. dyspareunia due to vaginal thrush.

Clinical examination can be an important part of the assessment of sexual problems. The main purpose may be to assess the part played by organic disease in any complaint but the examination may also serve to educate the patient or to increase his/her sexual confidence (e.g. in vaginismus).

Investigations

The urine should be tested for glucose in all men presenting with secondary impotence or late-onset ejaculatory problems. Superficial dyspareunia in women may indicate the need for a variety of tests such as a vaginal swab or full genitourinary screening. Ultrasound or laparoscopy may be needed in the assessment of deep dyspareunia. Measurements of erectile function such as nocturnal tumescence studies, measurement of penile blood pressure and blood-flow, and more invasive procedures such as arteriography, intracavernosal injections of smooth muscle relaxants and peripheral nerve conduction tests are also specialist techniques.

It is customary to measure serum testosterone, FSH, LH and prolactin levels in men complaining of loss of sexual interest or erectile difficulties but the results are seldom outside normal limits.

Treatment

The general principles of treating sexual dysfunctions include:

1. Consider treating the couple irrespective of which partner presents
2. Define the problem and what the couple would like to change
3. Aim to reduce sexual anxiety by education and 'permission giving'

which may modify unhelpful attitudes. Fear of unwanted pregnancy may be a source of anxiety and contraceptive counselling may prove to be therapeutic

4. Facilitate communication between the partners
5. Encourage new behaviour which will give mutual pleasure to the couple
6. Specific problems may need specific treatment programmes, e.g. vaginismus
7. Tackle more difficult interpersonal or intrapersonal problems if they appear to be 'blocking' progress.

Management of specific problems

Lack of sexual interest

The management of this problem will be the management of the underlying cause. Endocrine abnormalities will be rare and more often the lack of desire is secondary to stress, fatigue, depression, physical illness, drugs (e.g. alcohol), other sexual dysfunctions or relationship difficulties.

Failure of sexual arousal

Failure of the lubrication/swelling response in women may result in dyspareunia, lack of enjoyment, resentment and withdrawal from sexual encounters. It may be treated as outlined in the general principles. It may be particularly beneficial to ban sexual intercourse for a limited time and to encourage graded pleasuring exercises as a substitute. Once sexual arousal and enjoyment has been re-established the couple may regain the confidence to enjoy intercourse again. Erectile impotence may be treated successfully by the same means, provided there is no major organic deficit. When organic factors predominate, the couple may decide to resort to physical treatments such as mechanical aids to erection, vascular surgery, penile prostheses, or intracavernous injections of smooth muscle relaxants (e.g. papaverine) as a last resort.

Vaginismus

This is an involuntary spasm of the pelvic floor muscles surrounding the lower part of the vagina which may prevent penetration or render it painful. It appears to be a learned response triggered by fear of penetration and although it is usually primary it may occur secondary to traumatic experiences such as childbirth. Treatment should aim to help the couple understand the nature of the problem (pictures and models are helpful). The woman should be encouraged to tackle the avoidance which is usually exhibited in any phobic condition and helped to embark on a system of graded exercises (using fingers or dilators) while learning progressively to gain control and relax the pelvic floor muscles. The partner's involvement and encouragement in treatment are usually beneficial. Operative treatment should be avoided.

Dyspareunia

The management involves treating the underlying cause.

Male dyspareunia is rare but may be caused by lacerations from over-sharp IUCD threads or from candidal or other infections which may also affect the female partner.

Female dyspareunia. The causes of female dyspareunia which may require treatment (in addition to failure of sexual arousal or vaginismus) include:

1. Vulval conditions: candidal vulvitis, herpes genitalis, urethral caruncle, Bartholinitis
2. Vaginal conditions: atrophic vaginitis, infective vaginitis (candidal or trichomonal), chemical vaginitis, vaginal scars
3. Pelvic conditions: cystitis, pelvic inflammatory disease, pelvic pain syndrome, endometriosis, fibroids, ovarian tumours, constipation, inflammatory bowel disease.

Orgasmic dysfunction

Many women do not experience orgasm during sexual intercourse. This knowledge may be therapeutic to women who regard themselves as 'inadequate' because they require additional clitoral stimulation to reach orgasm. The capacity to experience orgasm may be helped by encouraging a couple to increase their sexual arousal (by 'super-stimulation') and by learning to relax and 'lose control' when high levels of sexual arousal are reached.

Premature ejaculation

Premature orgasm is only complained of in the male as his orgasm usually terminates sexual intercourse. Anxiety reduction and re-education to control the ejaculatory reflex are the basis for most therapeutic approaches.

SUMMARY

Sexual problems are common and may be presented to doctors overtly or covertly. The patient will choose to present their problem because she/he believes the doctor has some expert interest, knowledge or skill and therefore problems are frequently aired in discussions about contraception, obstetrics or gynaecology.

Concerned attention by the doctor at the first presentation may need to be followed by referral to a specialist but this should not be the initial response. The treatment of some conditions will be within the scope of the primary care doctor.

Appendix I

Obstetric terms and definitions

Amniotomy. Surgical rupture of the membranes to induce or enhance labour.

Android pelvis. A funnel-shaped male-type pelvis with diameters which decrease from above downwards.

Antepartum haemorrhage. Bleeding from the birth canal in the period from the 28th week of gestation to the birth of the baby.

Asynclitism. Tilting of the fetal head in labour so that the anterior or posterior parietal bone presents.

Attitude of the fetus. Relationship of fetal head and limbs to the fetal trunk, usually flexion.

Bregma. Anterior fontanelle.

Brow. The part of the fetal head between the root of the nose and the anterior fontanelle.

Caput succedaneum. Oedema from obstructed venous return in the fetal scalp caused by pressure of the head against the rim of the cervix or birth canal.

Cephalhaematoma. Collection of blood beneath the periosteum of a skull bone, limited to that bone by periosteal attachments.

Cervical dystocia. Difficult labour due to failure of the cervix to dilate, in spite of adequate uterine contractions.

Chloasma. The brown pigmented facial mask of pregnancy.

Couvelaire uterus. The uterus appears purple due to haemorrhage within its musculature, and occurs with severe placental abruption.

Crowning of the head. Phase in the second stage of labour when a large segment of the fetal scalp is visible at the vaginal orifice, the perineum being distended and the anus dilated.

Engagement. Engagement occurs when the widest diameters of the presenting part have passed through the pelvic inlet.

Erythroblastosis. Haemolytic disease of the newborn usually due to rhesus antibodies.

Fontanelle. Space at the junction of three or more skull bones, covered only by a membrane and skin.

Fourchette. The fold of skin formed by merging of the labia minora and labia majora posteriorly.

Funnel pelvis. (See Android pelvis.)

Hyaline membrane. A homogeneous membrane lining the alveoli, alveolar ducts, and respiratory bronchioles, and an important cause of death in premature infants.

Hydrops fetalis. Gross oedema of fetal subcutaneous tissues together with ascites, pericardial and pleural effusions, usually due to erythroblastosis.

Kernicterus. Yellow staining of the baby's brain due to high blood levels of bilirubin causing severe neurological damage or death.

Lie of the fetus. Relationship of the long axis of fetus to the long axis of the uterus, usually longitudinal, but can be transverse or oblique.

Linea nigra. Brown or black pigmented line in the middle of the abdominal wall during pregnancy.

Lochia. The discharge from the uterus during the puerperium, initially red, then yellow, then white.

Lower uterine segment. The thin expanded lower portion of the uterus which forms in the last trimester of pregnancy.

Moulding. Alteration in shape and diameters of the fetal head during labour (the fontanelles and sutures permit the force of contractions to compress the head against the bony pelvis and adapt its shape to that of the birth canal).

Naegle's rule. To estimate the probable date of confinement add 9 months and 7 days to the first day of the menstrual cycle (correction is required if cycle not 28 days).

Neonatal death. A liveborn infant who dies within 28 days of birth.

Obstructed labour. There is no descent of the presenting part in the presence of good contractions.

Operculum. The plug of mucus that occludes the cervical canal during pregnancy.

Pawlik's grip. Suprapubic palpation with the outstretched hand to identify the presenting part of the fetus, its position, flexion, and its station.

Pelvic brim or inlet. The plane of division between the true and false pelvis. The plane passes from the upper border of the symphysis pubis, along the pubic crest to the iliopectineal eminence, then to the sacroiliac joint, along the wings of the sacrum to the centre of the sacral promontory.

Pelvic outlet. Runs from beneath the symphysis pubis along the ischiopubic ramus to the ischial tuberosity along the sacrotuberous ligament to the fifth sacral vertebra.

Pelvimetry. Measurement of the size of the pelvis.

Perinatal mortality. Stillbirths plus first week deaths expresed per 1000 total births.

Placenta accreta. Absence of decidua basalis, so that the chorionic villi are attached to uterine muscle.

Placenta circumvallata. Placenta with a double fold of amnion forming a ring on the fetal surface some distance in from the edge of the placenta.

Placenta increta. Chorionic villi are in the uterine muscle.

Placenta percreta. The villi are through the uterine muscle.

Placenta succenturiata. There is one or more accessory lobe of the placenta.

Position of the fetus. The relationship of a defined area on the presenting part (called the denominator) to the quadrants of the maternal pelvis.

Presenting part. That part of the fetus felt on vaginal examination.

Prolonged pregnancy. A pregnancy that lasts longer than term (37–42 completed weeks).

Puerperium. The period during which the reproductive organs return to their prepregnant condition (usually regarded as an interval of 6 weeks after delivery).

Show. A discharge of mucus and blood at the onset of labour when the cervix dilates and the operculum (cervical mucus plug) falls out.

Sinciput. That part of the fetal head in front of the anterior fontanelle.

Spalding's sign. Overlapping of the fetal skull bones, seen radiographically after fetal death.

Station. The level of the presenting part within the mother's pelvis (the ischial spines are the reference points on vaginal examination).

Symphysiotomy. Division of the pubic symphysis to enlarge the diameters of the bony pelvis.

Third degree tear. A perineal laceration passing through the anal sphincter.

Vasa praevia. Fetal vessels lying in the membranes in front of the presenting part (there must be an associated velamentous insertion of the cord, succenturiate lobe, or bipartite placenta).

Velamentous insertion. The umbilical cord inserts onto the membranes over which the vessels course to reach the fetal surface of the placenta.

Vernix caseosa. Produced by sebaceous glands and prevents waterlogging and maceration of the fetal skin by the amniotic fluid.

Vertex. The area between the anterior and posterior fontanelles and the parietal eminences.

Wharton's jelly. The mucoid connective tissue supporting the umbilical cord vessels.

Appendix II

Risk factors in obstetrics

General factors	Age less than 18 years Age more than 36 years Nullipara of 35 or more Parity greater than 4
Menstrual history	Last period more than 2 weeks uncertain Pill stopped within 3 months of last period Cycle length before last period more than 30 days Intrauterine device in situ Vaginal bleeding since last period
Previous obstetric history	Stillbirth or neonatal death Small baby, less than 2.5 kg Large baby, more than 4.0 kg Fetal congenital abnormality Significant antibodies (defined by haematologist) Hypertension or proteinuria Eclampsia Two or more legal abortions (less than 13 weeks) Two or more miscarriages (less than 13 weeks) Late miscarriage or legal abortion (13 weeks or more) Preterm delivery (less than 37 weeks) Cervical suture Caesarean section, hysterotomy, or myomectomy Postpartum haemorrhage or manual removal of placenta

Labour less than 2 hours
Labour more than 12 hours
Operative vaginal delivery
Postnatal depression

Maternal health

Relevant medical condition
Pelvic abnormality (including fibroids)
Smoking more than 10 per day at booking
Social factors
Problems with housing
Family history of diabetes
Family history of congenital abnormality
Haemaglobinopathy
Risk of transmissible viral factors
Drinking more than 10 units alcohol per week at booking
Current drug abuse by woman or partner
Not fluent in English

Booking examination

Blood pressure more than 140/90
Proteinuria
Weight more than 90 kg
Weight less than 45 kg
Height less than 1.52 m
Cardiac murmur
Uterus large or small for dates
Other pelvic or abdominal mass
Blood group rhesus negative

City and Hackney District Health Authority system (from Carroll et al 1988 Journal of Obstetrics and Gynaecology 8: 222–227).

Appendix III

The fetal skull

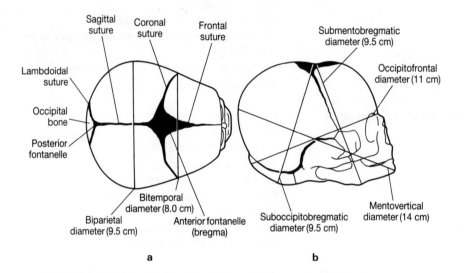

Fig. III
Frontal suture—between the two frontal bones
Coronal suture—between the frontal and parietal bones
Sagittal suture—between the two parietal bones
Lambdoidal suture—between the occipital bone and the parietal and temporal bones.

Anterior fontanelle (bregma)—large diamond-shaped depression where the frontal, coronal and sagittal sutures meet. Closes at 18 months of age.
Posterior fontanelle—smaller triangular-shaped depression where the sagittal suture meets the lambdoidal sutures.

Diameters of the fetal skull
Biparietal diameter: 9.5 cm (vertex presentation)
Submentobregmatic: 9.5 cm (face presentation)
Occipitofrontal: 11 cm (deflexed head, usually occipitoposterior)
Mentovertical: 14 cm (brow presentation)
Suboccipitobregmatic: 9.5 cm (vertex presentation).

Appendix IV

Diameters of the normal female pelvis

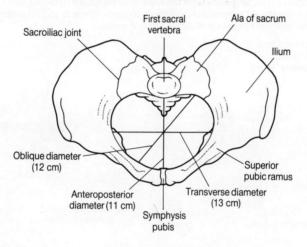

Fig. IVA: The pelvic brim
The outline of the brim follows the upper border of the first sacral vertebra, the alae, the sacroiliac joint, the ilium, the superior pubic ramus and the symphysis pubis.

Anteroposterior diameter: 11 cm
Oblique diameter: 12 cm
Transverse diameter: 13 cm.

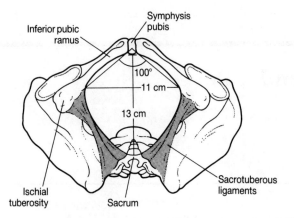

Fig. IVB: The pelvic outlet

The boundary of the outlet passes from the symphysis pubis, down the inferior rami of the pubic bones to the ischial tuberosities, and then obliquely upwards and posterior along the sacrotuberous ligaments to the tip of the fifth sacral vertebra.

Anteroposterior: 13 cm
Transverse: 11 cm
Oblique diameter: 12 cm.

Appendix V

The obstetric flying squad

Obstetric flying squads were pioneered by E. F. Murray in Newcastle in the 1930s, and comprise an obstetrician, midwife and anaesthetist with the necessary equipment to resuscitate a woman prior to transfer to hospital.

Some 30% of calls are for intrapartum problems and 50% for PPH or retained placenta. Removal of a retained placenta is one of the few operative procedures now performed at home.

Indications to summon the flying squad:

1. Intrapartum haemorrhage
2. Eclampsia or severe pre-eclampsia
3. Postpartum haemorrhage
4. Retained placenta
5. Neonatal apnoea.

Appendix VI

Normal values in pregnancy

Haemoglobin concentration:	12 weeks	12.0 g/dl
	36 weeks	11.1 g/dl
White cell count:	12 weeks	8.1×10^6
	36 weeks	10.2×10^6
Packed cell volume		< 0.35
Platelets		$< 175 \times 10^6$
ESR		44–114
Serum urate:	32 weeks	< 0.35 mmol/l
Serum urate:	36 weeks	< 0.40 mmol/l
Serum glucose (fasting)		< 5.5 mmol/l
Serum glucose (random)		< 8.7 mmol/l
Glomerular filtration rate		170 ml/minute
24 hour urinary protein		< 0.3 g/24 hours

Appendix VII

Partograms—the graphic description of labour

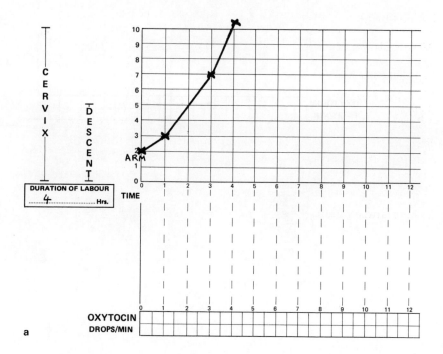

a

Partograms showing **a**. normal labour and **b**. inefficient uterine action corrected with oxytocin, overleaf

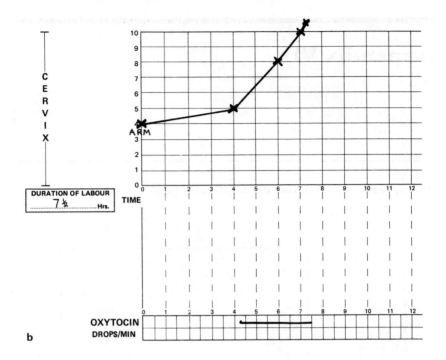

b

Index